You're Number 1!
Ben Harris

Books by Ben Harris

Fiction:

- The adventure of Harry and George in the illusion of time
- The Little girl and the tiger cub
- Wrath of the Empire

Non-fiction:

- You're number 1
- Diet 66

If you're a passionate reader and interested in becoming a beta reader with free access to early releases, then reach out by email. I would love to have you on board.

For more information

Contact: BenjaminHarris@gmx.com

First published in Great Britain in 2020 by Ben Harris

2 3 4 5 6 7 8 9 10

First printed and bound in Great Britain in 2020 by Ben Harris

ISBN 9798613598847

The first book by Ben Harris

"Very little is needed to make a happy life; it is all within yourself, in your way of thinking." – Marcus Aurelius

Introduction

"You're Number 1!" was written to help people learn about some basic areas of life that they may not have learnt in school, from family, or anywhere else. It all relates to you and the areas of your life you may want to work on, for you to become whatever you want in life; for you to put yourself first for once, look after yourself, and achieve anything you could ever dream of.

Before I get into the part where I tell you about me and who I want to acknowledge, I thought I would first dedicate the book to anyone out there who has lost somebody in any way–if they were lost, their life has changed, and everything stopped being the way it was after people moved on–if they have passed away or passed by. This is for anyone who is alone, lost, hurt, broken, down, out, upset, depressed, unhappy, self-harming, suicidal, or feeling incomplete. I hope this finds you and helps you to find companionship, but most importantly, yourself. I hope it helps you to heal, get up, wake up, find happiness, save yourself, and become complete. At the very least, if there is no one out there for you and this doesn't help, then I will be there for you; get in touch. I will do anything I can to help and support you to a better life. It is what you deserve; it is what everyone deserves.

In writing and completing this book, I did something that I always wanted to do–to be an author. A lot of people want to, but may not actually get to start or even finish it. In my opinion, it is no easy feat and has opened my eyes and lead me to having great respect for anyone who has already completed and/or published a book. Before writing this book, I had two previous attempts, which so far have yet to be completed, and both are still works in progress. I will eventually return to them and I will complete them. So, how did I get here? How did I produce this book? What inspired me?

It all started with a documentary about an American author, entrepreneur, life coach and philanthropist. Well, that wasn't the real start, as there was a bit more before that; but I'm not ready to tell you the bit before just yet. So, after watching the documentary, I went on to read his books. In doing so, I learned that the top CEOs in the world read 60 books a year on average, amongst other things. I then went on to read more than 60 books that year. As a result, I covered a wide range of topics and learnt a lot of things. I became obsessed with reading and then decided to go back to writing. Afterwards, I produced this book, bringing together some of the key points I had learned from the vast range of information I gathered.

In reading some of the books, I came across something in life which I didn't realise I had been looking for, something that I believe everyone wants and everyone deserves–happiness. I would go as far to say I reached a point of euphoric happiness without anything stimulating it except my own mind. No external factors affected it at all; so I could have it whenever I wanted, especially since I had taken full control over my mind and emotions. I still, to this day, find it quite unreal and will try to cover it the best way I can in this book and to share it with as many people as possible. I still learn new things all the time that can help, but I am not by any means perfect. So, it can be sometimes good to revisit methods if needed. Not every chapter in this book may fully hit the point of that topic, but they may cover other things you may find useful in your life and help to make little things a lot better.

I don't want to go as far as labelling this a self-help book, but I'm sure I learned a few things during my times of reading over 60 books that year, and I am still reading. I also don't see anything wrong with labelling it a self-help book, even if there is a bit of stigma attached to them. I know people who have been in bad places with their mindset and turned to medication, alcohol, and counselling, and I have even seen the worst that can happen with someone taking their own life. I didn't take or needed any of that because as far as I'm concerned, if you read a book that helps you, then that has got to be the best possible solution to your challenges. I look at it as education more than anything, as you may not know simple things in life which you could learn from a book that could make your life amazing.

I find that just reading alone can help, as the mind is being used and is learning, which gives it even more purpose, on top of the fundamental and amazing things it can already do. If you do find this book helpful in any way to your journey to achieving happiness and a better-quality family life, money, sleep etc., then I would love to hear about it. So, please get in touch through any of the options below. I hope you find this book to be worthy of your time and that the message I aim to deliver comes across the way it was intended. I hope it helps everyone who reads it, in the way that information in it has helped me.

I find in reading a book, you can read someone else's thoughts, views, opinions, and knowledge. You are then able to take that information and read it as though you are giving advice to yourself, which can help you to put it in practice. This is done instead of just listening to someone else say it to you, although people tend to listen if they want to.

So, I guess you picked this up because you wanted to. As such, please enjoy and take from it whatever you need. Although I struggled with previous ones, this one I completed in less than one percent of the time that I spent on the others, and I credit that to the "10x rule," which made me switch my focus from writing and completing one book to having a goal of writing and completing 10 books. In doing so, my original goal of one book was completed in a matter of a few months rather than dragged out over years like the previous two. I now also have the focus and the drive to go on and complete the others and aim for that target of 10.

If you find this does help you in any way and you know someone that may benefit from it, then please pass it on. I would rather it helped someone if they needed it over them not reading it because they didn't or couldn't buy it. So, by all means, share it, lend it, or even give it away (even though I would prefer they purchased it as it will help me to work less and spend more time writing and producing more work like this). However, my sole aim is really to help people more than profit from it—in order to give back, to reduce the negativity in the world, and to reduce the stress and unhappiness in the world by helping people to find themselves.

Whatever happens to you in your life, I wish you all the best. I hope that you enjoy the journey and I hope that you travel along that journey for as long as possible. If I ever get to meet you, then I would love to hear your story, hear about things you have learned in life, and share a smile and a laugh. Maybe one day, you might even write a book, and if you do, then send me a link to it as I would love to read it. Approach this book with an open mind if you can. Let yourself change to whatever it is you want to be and let yourself be great. Don't go in with high expectations, go in with an empty mind and take out anything you want. Take out the guidance that you feel will help you and use it for a better life. If you don't get anything from it, then I'm sorry. Maybe try it again if it wasn't too painful. Alternatively, let me know, so I could recommend some other great books that have helped me in the past. Whatever the result, be you, be what you want, when you want, but be it with happiness, values, and dreams in place. Enjoy watching the world go by and enjoy your journey through life.

Acknowledgements:

Thank you to my daughter. You inspired me so much and motivated me so much and gave me so much purpose and value. I love you with all my heart.

Thank you, Mum and Dad, for showing me values and teaching me to work hard for what I want. My sister for supporting me during hard times. Gran for showing that happiness can still be there no matter what your age.

Thank you to the people that supported me with this project and motivated me to complete it.

Thank you to anyone who has picked this book up and spent some of their time, a part of their life, to sit down and read it. It means a lot to me. I hope it has helped you.

Chapters

Chapter 1-Find Yourself and Balance Your Life

A few years back, my life got a bit flipped on its head and I came to realise that I had lost myself and my identity because of another person. I allowed that person to take control a bit and forced her ideas on me, therefore, taking over my life. That was a mistake, and it was my own fault for letting it happen. When she left, it took me a fair bit of time and soul searching to realign myself, and I eventually got back on track to how I wanted my life to be rather than how someone else wanted it to be. I started reading, which was something I always wanted to do more of, and it became something that I still love to this day. It helped me to learn, grow, and educate myself to a level I could never have dreamed of reaching. Most of all, it taught me a lot of things in life that I was never taught in school; such as how to handle money, investing, relationships, business, parenting, and happiness. These were all things I needed as I had been through a hard time, and I am pretty certain I even suffered some post-traumatic stress–a real level of sadness–although I don't believe I was depressed. I definitely felt lost, lacked direction, had lost someone I loved, and it hurt; the feeling of heartbreak is like nothing else. So, I needed help, but I didn't turn to alcohol, drugs, counselling or anything like that. I turned to books and good old exercise–both of which have helped me to find my direction and got me back on track to living my life's mission. I am able to be the best dad I can be to my daughter, be there for others who need help, and I have secured a stable financial future for myself and my family. I have learnt a lot and want to share it with you in this book, along with some further reading that has taken my life to a great level.

The most important thing is to be honest with yourself, find out who are you, what you want, your values, your missions, where you are going with your life, and what is important to you. So, that's what we are going to look at. To find yourself, you have to ask yourself those pertinent questions. However, there's more to it than that, because if there wasn't, then I wouldn't have had a book to write. Think about the people you are around and how they live their lives; how do they influence you? Do you act like them? Do you learn from them? Do you do things they do? Or is it the other way around; are they like you? Think about who you are and what you do, no matter your age, then make your own choices, think for yourself, be you, and don't just live your days doing the same old things, stuck in your routine. Think about what choice you want to make and live every day for what you want.

Think about taking each day as it comes. Anything in the past that has happened doesn't matter because it's gone; so, don't let it affect you. The future hasn't even happened yet (I quote from Back to the Future 3, where this is the main point to the story); hence, there is no need to worry about it, especially since you have no control over it. So, live for the day you're in, keep your focus, and if someone is talking to you, then listen to them, maintain eye contact, and fully engage with what they are saying. It might be important and could actually help you. They have gone out of their way to talk to you, so respond, stop drifting off, and when you sit down to eat something, don't rush it, enjoy it.

When you're driving down the road breaking the speed limit, overtaking people to get somewhere quicker, to save 10 minutes max, consider the fact that you are putting people's lives at risk. It is best to slow down a bit, as it's not worth it. There are enough hours in the day to do everything you need to do and if there isn't, then it's because you haven't planned it properly. Therefore, you need to make a better plan for your day, month and even year. It doesn't matter if it has to be done today, tomorrow, or next week. As long as you have it planned, then you don't need to be rushing around for your boss, to get home to a partner, meet up with friends, or for anyone else.

 A lot of things you do are they for you, for other people, or does it relate back to you somehow? Are you really doing it for you? We will look at discovering your goals, your mission, your values, and finding happiness. (We will cover values and missions further, in another chapter). Once you have achieved these things, then it gives you purpose and makes life worth living, and that's what I want you to think about at this time. Think about you and about what you want and why you are here? Really, why are we here? Well, only you can know the answer for yourself because we are all here for different reasons. For me, I know why I'm here and my purpose, so I want to help you find yours. Everyone's reason is different, and if someone you know can't find theirs, then maybe this book can help them. So, once you finish reading it, then maybe you can help them. Along with your guidance and support (that's once you have your values, your mission, and everything else), you can help others. They might not want to listen to you, and I wouldn't recommend preaching or forcing it on anyone. But if you're happy and enjoying your life, then people may ask you how and what you did to get to where you are, and you can certainly share with them. Having a purpose and a mission and helping others can bring you further happiness.

Before we even touch on those points, think about what you
have. A lot of books will speak about gratitude and appreciating
what you have. Well, they are right! It's important. If you don't
appreciate what you have and are not grateful, then you are not
going to be happy. It's as simple as that. If you want to be happy,
you need to appreciate every little thing; even if it's the sun
coming up or going down, the rain falling from the sky, the cars
on the road, the traffic, or whatever. As much as people hate it,
the people we pass on the road and in traffic are going
somewhere and they will probably be serving us in a shop,
restaurant, or could be the nurse or doctor who will help us in the
hospital. Be grateful for everything and take a moment every day
to appreciate things and people. Be grateful for family, friends,
and having a roof over your head. Because if you don't, you
won't be happy; not all the time, just temporarily. If you want to
be happy, you will have to be happy with what you have. Maybe
even give back or help others. It can contribute to making other
people's lives better.

If you were to spend £5 on yourself, it might make you happy
for the day. But if you gave £5 to charity or someone in the street
that needed it, then it would bring you happiness for a much
longer period. It can be that it's helped them in a good way. You
won't know for a fact, but you will benefit from the act of giving
back, and it will make you feel a better person. Consider giving
back, appreciating what you have; not thinking about what you
want, what you think you might need, or what you could have.
Some of the happiest people on the planet have very little.

I can't imagine that anyone who has everything is truly happy.
You still get very wealthy and very famous people that take their
lives; so, why aren't they happy? What causes them to do that?
We will touch on that mental health, pure health, things that can

affect us, such as alcohol and substances, and things that make us unhappy. What makes you unhappy? Is it something you want in your life, something you need, or something that affects you? Think about what bothers you and what your real problems are. Your problem may not come from little things–it could be something that happened a week ago, a month, or years and years ago, and you might still be taking it out on other people. It could be ongoing and could have bothered you for a long time. It could affect your relationships. Maybe you need to get rid of what's really bothering you. List everything that bothers you in life– actually get a notepad and get it down on paper. Think why and does it matter and can you eliminate those things and not let it bother you? For example, traffic. Is it your own fault? Did you leave the house late? Did you fail to plan out your day? Take ownership and eliminate the problem with simple methods suggested later in the book.

Let's get to a point when we can be okay. We can really be good people or even great ones. So, look at the opposite–what makes you happy–and get it down on paper. Do you come home every night and watch T.V.? Does that make you happy or are you just stuck in a routine? Is it just that you need rest and then you end up not moving or getting anything done? Do you drink four to five cups of coffee a day or are you stuck in a routine? Has it just snowballed? Is it routine and excessive consumption? Think about doing the things you want to do rather than taking the easy route of not thinking and being on autopilot. If you don't want that coffee, then don't make it. Stop and think. Before you do anything, stop and think. Do I want this or is it just a habit? Is it a routine? Maybe I will have something different? Then this can happen with anything and everything. Are you happy going to work? Do you need to go to work? What other options are there? Can you retrain your behaviours? Could you change your job, read a book, and learn something new, do an evening course, or start your own business?

How are your relationships? Are you happy? Does it make you happy? Do you give happiness and receive from the relationship? You should be happy first, then express it in the relationship. Don't enter one looking for happiness because if you leave it, then you could be in trouble. Find happiness first, then share it– take it into the relationship. Enjoy it and share it equally. Find someone that is happy as then they can bring happiness too. If not, then you may have a battle on your hands. Your partner may be sucking the happiness out of you–like good vs evil. Make Happiness your priority every day. The first thing to do is to make sure you enter your day with it and then share it with everyone–your family, friends, and your kids.

So, what if your kids are jumping on the bed? Will it make you happy to shout at them? No, it will make you miserable. Do you care if it breaks? Probably a little bit. Stop caring about the money aspect; let go of that. There's a good chance it won't break. So, let go and just be happy. That little thing is contributing to you being unhappy. If it breaks, then you may have to replace it. It will cost you some money, but guess what? You can earn more money to pay for it. You work, you get paid, and then you get paid the following month, and then the one after. So, you can pay for it. The money will keep coming. But that moment of misery that you have chosen to have, you can't get that moment back; it's gone. Let it happen, let go, forget fear–that will bring you sadness and misery. The fear of anything can give us a sense of caution and worry. It can make us sad, angry, or even shout at the ones we love. It's okay. It's okay if you are people will forgive you. It's the same with sadness. It's okay if you are. It's okay to express your emotions, to let it out and to let it go. Sometimes it's best to save it and let it out at the right time, when the kids don't see it. Wait until you are in the gym and you can take it out on a punching bag or the treadmill, but don't overdo it. We will touch on the necessity of fitness later.

Find what's true to you and what makes you happy. Does going to the gym make you happy or are you doing it because you feel pressured to go? Does it make you happy to read a book, but you never do it? Get it written down. Get on paper a list of the things you like, the things that make you happy, the things that don't make you happy. Then get rid of those ones or get your mindset around them and don't let them bother you anymore. For things that make you happy, how do they make you feel that way? How often can you do them? How often do you just appreciate waking up and having breakfast with your kids and just sit there enjoying the moment? Maybe just not cleaning the kitchen for ten minutes and spending some time watching cartoons with the kids. That would be more fun. I think sometimes as adults we forget how good a cartoon can be or playing toys with our kids. Or how often do you do things that are relaxing and enjoyable? Get it all down on paper. Get a clear insight of you and only you and what you want and what's good for you and only you. What is life about? What is it about for you and for what you want? What's the meaning of it and the purpose of it? Because once you find yours and you're in that good place, then you will be happy. You can help yourself, and you can help others.

Remember, if they don't want help, then it's no good trying to help them if they won't want it. If they are not in the right mindset, then you can't bring them happiness. Honestly, they must be ready emotionally to listen. Wait until the moment is right. People will listen to themselves a lot more than they will listen to others. But don't let this affect you, don't let their mindset change yours. Let your happy mindset change everyone else.

Take some time away from the family, friends, partner, or kids (don't leave them on their own, though). So, go for a walk, go for a drive, maybe even sit on the toilet; stay there for a few extra minutes and you may only need a few minutes. Maybe you need half a day or even six months or more to think about what makes you happy. You may even have to try a few things out. There is probably a lot of things out there that you haven't even tried, and it could be sports, recreational activities, leisure, or different types of work. Whatever it is, it could take time. Some people go their whole life not knowing what they want to do for work or what they enjoy in life; so, make time for it. It should be your life's mission to find out what makes you tick, as when you do, things get a little bit better and life is a little bit sweeter.

How can you then create a balance of life covering family, health, fitness, and work? There's plenty of tools online, including the wheel of life. I believe the wheel of life is commonly used in counselling and may even originate from Buddhism, which uses a similar tool. It is mainly used to find a balance and have a prosperous life. Rearrange and change it to suit you, as it's your life and should be laid out how you want to live it. I suggest you look at areas you want to work on and improve on. However, you don't even need a wheel. You could just have a list and you can include things such as family, health, career, personal development, money, relationships, and even leisure activities. You can then rate them on a scale from one to ten. Rate each area on how you perceive your life—one being bad and ten being good. You should base it purely on your opinion and consider every area of each category. Set it out just as a guide and use it as a tool to rate your life and establish where you're low and where you're high. It can help you to identify what you want to work on and improve, as well as areas where you might be excelling. It can even contribute to your plan. It can be a good way of measuring success and is commonly used by successful people. It also eliminates focusing on other people and how they live their life and helps you to live by your own standards.

You might not have the same category as other people, as you may not have much family or money might not matter to you (although there is a good chance you need it, even if it's just for food and rent). But the key thing is to make sure it's built around you and what you want. Create a list, have it in a notebook or paper diary. Forget the phone. We spend too much time on them as it is already; unless you really must, and it works for you to use it. Review your list or cycle, not every six months, but as much as possible. If you can do it daily, then great; but weekly or monthly should be sufficient. Rate each area out of 10. Aim to build them all up to 10 or as close as you can. But most importantly, make sure there is a balance and aim to increase the numbers, by increasing time with family, or decreasing time at work, the money you spend, or money you earn. If you are scoring 7-8 across the board, then you are in a good place. If you have a mix of fours, eights, and so on, then you may have some work to do; unless you look at it and are happy with it. That could be how you want to live your life–there's not really a wrong or right. The only right is what you want and what will make you happy. It's just guidance, and it's there for you to use as a tool and get the most you can out of it. So, use your diary or pad, and decide how often you review it. Maybe even do it alongside your goals in a subsequent chapter.

But if you do use it, make sure it works for you and you get something out of it; don't just use it for the sake of it. You can include all types, including sleep, exercise, diet, happiness or your home (maybe the cleanliness). That can all contribute to your happiness. A dirty home and bad environment won't make you happy, so put it on there. This can help you establish finding yourself and what you want, finding a good balance, help to cover each area of your life, and be more of a complete person. You may be working too much or not enough, or too much time is spent with your family. This may cause you to have time management issues. That might be the case and that might be okay with you. But remember to use the tool to help you and how you want to use it.

It is advised to have a daily routine. Have your goals listed and your successes? What did you achieve from your list? Was it from the to-do list? Was it from your goals or your dreams list? What works? What have you done? You can review it for the week. It can help you plan out your week. You can look at changes on your scale and see how you're progressing. You might find yourself improving in one area and a deteriorate in other areas. But that's what this does; it shows it and helps you to identify it. Life can be a challenge–looking after yourself, your kids, your family, juggling it with work, the gym, and everything else. Don't create limits. Use this tool to help you see where you can improve, and keep moving forward to improve and become the best that you can be. In the words of Rocky: "It's not about how hard you can hit, it's about how hard you can get hit and keep moving forward." Lay it out, write it down, whether you do it on a wheel or list is up to you. You can get templates online that you can print out. I prefer a notebook and writing it down and taking ownership of it. There is some good stuff online, so by all means, have a look even if it's just to get an idea. Try my route but consider what works for you as that will always be the best option; and only you will know what works for you. This will help you to find fulfilment and do what matters to you and will help you to find happiness through a stable balance in life. Think about what makes you happy (we will explore that more in Chapter 2), get that balance and focus on the things that make you happy, move towards them, and there's no reason those goals can't be achieved today.

Whatever has happened in the past has gone, and whatever happens in the future, you have no control over. So, focus on right now and what you can do right now to make you happy. The first thing you should do when you wake up is to clear the cobwebs in your mind and forget everything–forget the routine, focus on what makes you happy, and what will help you to enjoy your day. It may be your routine, but you have no control over that. Maybe even create a to-do list. What do you want to get out of your day? What will make you happy? What will be a success? What will you enjoy? What will be great about it? If it means staying in bed, then fine. If it's getting up and having a coffee, great. Make sure you are not overstretching yourself; life should be easy, and it should be great; not because of money or family, but a great balance of many things.

Too much of anything is not good for you. I have a great life now because I strike that balance. I've suffered in the past with too much work and not enough family time, or not enough money, and so on. So, enjoy what you have, one day at a time. There is no tomorrow; only right now. Plan ahead but remember Mike Tyson once said: "Everyone has a plan until they get knocked out." (I love to quote famous sayings and will drop a few more throughout the book.) Find your happiness, work on it, and move forward with it. Let go, enjoy where you are, and life will be okay. No other moment matters than now. Take life as it comes and roll with it. You don't have to keep pushing back; you can roll with the punches for a change and take things as they come by going with the flow of it. Sometimes it's not worth thinking about things that will cause you pain or dwelling on them. Instead, take some time to sit down, think about it, and make sense of it. Maybe even talk it out with someone to help you find out what it is that bothers you and get an understanding of it. Then move on, work on those areas that matter to you and improve and be as good as you want to be. Let that be your focus and let that consume your time. Give yourself a healthier balance to life by driving towards a better you and the you that you want to be. List out the key areas and maybe even lay out the priorities of where you would like to improve the most. For example, you may be low in one area, but you might be fine with it being low. What matters is that you know where you want to improve, then think about how you want to improve, what you can do to make those areas and your life better and to make you happier. This is just the start. From here, we will go on to making goals, finding your purpose, going over the different areas in life and how they can be improved, and then taking action to get everything happening. We will also get you moving forward and get you to the point of fully enjoying and making the most of your life and living your dreams.

Chapter 2–Values, Missions, Dreams and breaking barriers

I once experienced the aftereffect of a horrendous situation in which I witnessed the aftermath of someone hanging themselves. It was, without a doubt, one of the toughest situations to experience and really quite traumatic, including the effect it had on the family. Having seen and been through such a situation and having worked with and known quite a lot of people over the years that have suffered from depression, anxiety, self-harm, and suicidal feelings, I made the decision that one of my missions would be to support and help people in this area. I took one of the worst things that have happened in my life and I used it to give me a mission and drive forward to help as many people as I can. I started by taking on working with a charity, volunteering my time to support people that needed it in this area, and still do, to this day. I have also experienced other situations that drove me with purpose and establish a mission to make the most from any bad situation, as it can give you real drive and real focus to move forward.

Values is a good place to start. This will help you to work towards your goals, so think about what you want in life, what's important to you, and what it is you value. What do you want to live for? Set out some values, such as who do you want to help, why you want to help them, what is it that you are grateful for, do you value time, money, family, work, etc. Get this set-out and in place. It will help you to live for something and define you as a person. It can also help you with goals and support you to help others, such as charities, with your time or money. This can help you to feel better about yourself and enjoy life; it feels better to give than to receive.

Okay, so let's look at the mission. You should ask yourself, what do I want to work towards? What are you about? What are you living for? The responses to these questions can be interchanged with your values. People talk about wanting to be happy, which shouldn't be a goal or a destination. Both life and happiness are a journey, not a destination–the destination is death, where you won't have time for either or you will have a lot of time for both or something. Who knows? The point is, you are here, and one day, you won't be. When you are gone, when you are in a different form of particle than your current state because you won't really die, you will just change form then. None of this will matter. Your choice is to be happy every day or to be unhappy every day–everything has an opposite, like yin and yang. So, pick; why would you pick to be unhappy and only you have control over it, no one else? So, then take control; be happy every day. You're the only person in control of that. Don't let anyone affect it. Take control of it. So, to get there, get in a good emotional state. Your mind may split into two parts–a conscious and subconscious part. You have control over part of your mind. The bit that takes over can work against you. So, get yourself in a good mindset and be happy. So, how do you do that? Think about your environment–a clean home over a dirty one, a well-lit one over a dim room, plants over no plants. Think about music; different types of music can affect your mind–think of what they play in supermarkets, coffee shops, gyms. They are all slightly different to set the mood. Music can uplift your mood, even provide motivation. The "Rocky" movies come to mind with the soundtrack laid over motivational scenes. Use everything you can that you have as a resource to make you happy. Why wouldn't you? This should be an absolute priority. We will touch on this more in the chapter on happiness. What else could you have for a mission, to raise good kids, exercise daily? Don't make it so much goal-based but more of a thing you can do daily and live for. Bring your lifecycle into it. It might be to focus on one of those areas.

Dreams are basically goals to work towards, but don't let that limit you. You should look at it as a dream and just set one or two that can be achieved. Have a list, a to-do list or a goal list. It could be for a house, car, kids, family, to go to Disney World (that one is on my list). Set goals as a daily goal, monthly goals, yearly goals, career goals, life goals. These can be set out and the smaller ones can build towards the longer ones. You can make the goals smart, specific–not just a nice car but what make, model, when do you want to have it by, and how much will it cost? Break that cost down on how long you will save for it or how you could work towards the monthly payments. It should also be measurable–measure it through outlining the time frame and how much it costs, and when you will get to it. Your goal should also be achievable–what will you do to achieve it? How will you fund the payments? Save money, work extra hours, work another job? Ensure that your goal is realistic–can you fund it within the set time frame with the amount you earn? Finally, let your goal have a suitable time frame–the date you want to achieve it by and plan out how much you need by that date. This is just an example. You may have to vary it for different goals, especially if no money is involved.

Get this all down on paper, plan it out, and write it down. Work out if there is an easier way of doing it. Will it affect your life cycle? Will it cost money which could affect your work hours, your family, your happiness, etc. If you want to save money, then should you be spending it and so forth. Lay the goal out

over short, medium, and long term–maybe one month, six
months or 12 months. For example, you want a £10,000 car and
can save that over a year. You can then set monthly goals based
on that amount. Can you get a loan and hit the goal today? Make
sure that happiness is at the top of the list. Will your goal make
you happier or less happy? A car, for example, might bring you
short-term happiness, but if you already have one that is paid off
and you upgrade or get a new one, then the monthly cost may
make you unhappy. Make sure you cover all the areas of your
lifecycle and they are relevant to you. Make sure they contribute
to your everyday happiness. If they don't, then get them off the
list. Find happiness first. Get that first. Start that right now, even
if you force yourself, even if you're fooling yourself, because
that is number one. You can trick your mind into healing your
body through the placebo effect. You can also trick your mind
into happiness. Just like the placebo effect will make you better,
tricking your mind into happiness will make you happy,
however, you do it. As Nike say in their slogan, "Just do it."

Be realistic and miserable or kid yourself and be happy. You
have control over your mind and everything else can fall in line.
Everything can be a goal. Tell people you're great. Don't let
other people's attitudes affect you. Let yours affect them. Don't
let negative news articles affect you. You don't even have to
watch them. You have no need to know about them.

We learn from others, and if that's what you see, then there's a
good chance that's what you will be. If it's raining outside,
what's the problem? No one goes out in it. People moan about it.
Forget that. Get out in it and enjoy it, like a kid who would jump
in the puddles. Do you remember what that was like? Why do we
stop doing stuff like that because we grow up and have to fall in
line with society or how people expect us to be? Because we all

want to be miserable and stop having fun? Hell no! Do what you want–remember, water brings life and life is what you want. If the streets are empty, then it's your street, you can do it. Be happy and enjoy. Some people might say it's impossible to be happy every day. Well, it is to them because that's what they think and that's what they believe, and they have full control over how their life will be. But if you have a different mindset, then you have a different life. Henry Ford once said: "If you think you can or think you can't, then you're right." So, if you think you can't be happy, then it isn't going to happen. Belief is everything.

Belief, or a dream, or imagining something, is always the first step of your journey. As for myself, I'm there. I honestly believe I have achieved it; I've had times when I have been 100% happy just because I wanted to be, without any external factors controlling it. Get it all down on paper–your missions, your values, and your dreams. Okay. So, my dream is to take my daughter to Disney World between the ages of eight and ten years old. So, I broke it down. Over the next 6-8 years, how much it would cost, divided by that time frame. I gave myself a savings target for each month, and then I knew the dream was in motion. A set account, named after the goal, was created, so I know I can get there, and I can achieve it. That's eight years away. Don't let time restrict you. It can be decades if it must be. Set the dream, get it down, and get the goal in motion. Plan it out. Do you want a car? How much is it? Break it down. Is it a house? Does it even cost money? Is it to spend more time with family? Can you start now? Think of them. Make a plan of doing something weekly or fortnightly together. That's a way of working to make the dream a reality. I could go to Disney World tomorrow, but going at age two for my daughter won't be the same as eight or 10 years old; so, I will wait. It's planned out and it will work. If I did it now, then I would have to come up with another goal to suit the time frame. Values should be from yourself, what's in yourself. It doesn't have to be planned out. Do you want to be a good person or make new friends? This is what you stand for and can be immediate, but still be aware of it. Write it in your notebook.

Who do you want to be? Your mission is what you are working for and towards. Do you want to be a good person? It doesn't have to be the dream, but kind of a goal. Have daily goals or monthly goals. Like I said, my goal is eight years away. I've planned it monthly, with money being saved each month. Get it all down on paper as goals, review it regularly, not quarterly. More than that, monthly at the minimum, maybe even weekly, especially if you have daily goals. Make it clear what you want and how you will get there. I do daily goals. Uncle G said, "So, I do it." I write books. I break it down into a daily goal–one to two hours or one to two thousand words, depending on how well prepped it is, and it works towards the end result of the book which is planned out based on the chapter count or the word count on the pre-planning of the content. That can hit a short-term goal of writing a book in a month, with medium-term of writing five to six books in six months, and 10 books in a year. It works. It's a true statistic that if you write down what you want to achieve with goals or even tasks or a to-do list, then you are more likely to achieve them. I can't remember what the stats or figures are specifically, but they are high. It's something like 33-66% more likely if you write it down. Now, if that is the true figure, then you increase your chances of success by a massive amount. Think about it: you want to buy a house but haven't written it down. Write it on paper; when do you want to achieve it by, how much money do you need? Work out the time frame, and plan out where you will get that amount from (whether it's a second job, overtime or money you already have coming in or money you are wasting on a sports or movie package or the latest phone). You then take that amount and set it aside in a separate account and then review the goal, the payment, the amount you have in your account each month, quarter, and year. It goes from a dream to real action in place and moving forward to the realisation of the dream.

Even if it was something simple as completing some daily tasks, such as cleaning the house, washing the car, and so on. You can create a list, plan it into your day, and then check them off one by one. You should be planning everything into your day, working out where every minute is going, including rest time. As you will need it, follow the plan, check it off, and see the results.

Life barriers exist that could prevent your goals, depending on your goals. But generally, you could lack time, might not have enough money, might not have support from your family, and may work too many hours. You can overcome these barriers and bring yourself back to the lifecycle. They can all interfere with each other, hence using the lifecycle balance chart to ensure you have a steady balance to your life. Make sure you have it all down on paper and review it weekly or even daily. What can you do? Well, if time is an issue, you can plan out your goals and then follow the plan to help overcome the time issue? Once things are planned out, you can look at how you can achieve them quicker in less time. So, for me, for example, writing this book. Rather than going straight to the laptop, I planned out what I wanted to write. I used a Dictaphone to record my thoughts, then typed it up afterward. This reduced all that thinking time and writer's block, enabling me to complete the book over a quicker period once the planning had been completed. If it was a fitness-related goal of getting in the gym and taking up exercise and you didn't have the time, you could ask a trainer to provide you with a short workout for beginners or look one up online you can do daily at home.

Let's look at career goals. If you wanted a change of a career but couldn't stop work to go to college, then can you do a course in the evening or do a distance learning course online? You might not be able to afford to do a course, so why not look at free courses, bursaries, or just reading an old-fashioned book. You get the idea? Don't let barriers be an excuse. Let it be what drives you to find a solution. What if you haven't got time to read? Then get an audiobook. Listen to it in the car or on the train to work. You can learn anything these days from economics, physics to programming. If you don't have the support of your family, then don't tell them about it. Find people that will support you. Network with people and find people with similar interests. Don't accept people telling you that you can't do it. You can do anything you want and it's better to try than to fail. Face the fear head-on. Not doing it is worse than failing, and you can learn from failing. Learn how not to do it, then tackle it in a different way. Work can take up most of your time and may not provide enough income. Are you working 40 hours and can't drop any? Do you have to work overtime and don't get paid extra? Then start to make the most of your time. If you become time rich, then you will become wealthy. It's not about the money. You will always have another paycheck coming, but you are always losing time. Work fast, get as much done as you can in your time, and free time up for other things, even if it's at home and not in the workplace. Can you clean the house in 30 minutes rather than 60? Can you cook dinner quicker and save yourself another 30 minutes? Do you waste time watching television when you could be learning, exercising, or working overtime? Are you in the gym for two hours when you could do one hour? Are you sleeping too much? Are you sleeping for 10 hours when all you need is eight? You could even have seven and still be okay and still be healthy. You could gain an extra seven to 21 hours a week from that alone? What would you do with all that time? Learn a language as you have always wanted to. What would you use it for? Is there any point? Make sure your goals are relevant to what you want? Write a book. Why just one? Why not 10? Get your balance right, get your time management right, plan out your day, and even add sleeping for seven to eight hours if you need to, then check it off if achieved.

The barrier of not having enough money is a reality to most. So, ask yourself, do you need it? Think about what you need and what you want. Food is a need, water is a need, clothing etc. Coffee, biscuits, five pairs of shoes are all wants in your life, i.e. not needed. So, if you don't have enough money and you are spending on things you don't need, can you reduce that amount? We will cover this more in the money section. But say you were running your own business and needed social media marketing. Can you do it yourself? Can you learn it from YouTube or a book? Do you have the time to do it? So, it comes back to that balance of money over time. Could you earn more money from working another job, overtime on your current job, or selling stuff online that you don't use anymore?

What about doubts? Do you doubt you can achieve these goals? How will you motivate yourself and how will you get in the right emotional state? Get yourself happy, find your right frame of mind, leave the house if you need to, and go and see people in your network. Break down that doubt and that fear and use it to motivate yourself. If you have a fear, then tackle it head-on because that fear is a sign; that fear is what will bring you success. Use all the resources you have–music, environment, get down to the gym and get the blood flowing, buy some fresh flowers for your house, or walk to the shop to buy them rather than driving.

Be positive around everyone and they will be positive in return. It's like the sea reflecting the sky. A clear blue sea gives us a clear blue sky, and a dark grey sea also reflects a dark grey sky. Don't lose time on planning. Do what you need, then move forward. Don't sit on it. Use the people around you. If you need someone to do something, then get them to do it for you. If you have a business and need a website, then consider if you are cash-rich or time rich. If cash, then pay someone to do it. If it is time, then get on YouTube or online books and learn it. Get that balance. Then consider if what you are doing is worth your time. Is it £10 per hour? Will it cost you more than if you paid someone? If it takes you three to four weeks to do it and you get someone to do it at a fraction of the cost of three to four weeks of your time, compared what you earn in that time. If you clean your car and it takes an hour at £10 per hour, yet the local car wash costs £5 and does it in 10 minutes, which is the better deal? Save 50 minutes of your life and the money you would have earned for that time.

So, are you a barrier to yourself? Do you waste time? Do you lack direction? Or do you drink, eat unhealthy foods causing you to be tired and fatigued? Do you have the wrong people around you? Can you change these things, get better food in you, drink less, stop taking drugs or medication that you don't need? Can you replace things, like alcohol with a nice soft drink, hot chocolate or coffee? Can you replace unhealthy foods with healthy snacks? Maybe replace drugs with unhealthy food and then work your way off that; it could be the lesser of two evils. Do you have the right mindset? Are you hung up on things that haven't worked or don't make you happy? How can you change this? Can you go back to that emotional state? Can you change the way you approach it? I'm sure it was Tony Robbins that said, "If you keep doing the same thing, then you will always get the same result." So, change your approach. If your website doesn't bring your business customers, then try Instagram–change your tact. If you write a book and it doesn't sell, change the cover, change the title, then send it back out there. Think about the way you do things, your working space. Is it calm? Are you better with people around you or on your own? Are you better off with music or without it? Then what type of music? Does jazz work or classical? Are you better at home or in a coffee shop? Do you have a diary for your day? Do you start with any exercise in the morning or late at night? How do you operate better? You might work better in the morning and need to get some rest at night, then come back at it fresh the next day. Sorry for all the questions, but they are there to get your mind thinking and are questions I want you to answer for yourself, as it may help you moving forward.

Remember to keep all these things in check with goals set in place, barriers laid out, and how you can beat them. With a to-do list, dreams laid out. Your support network, your lifecycle and the perfect working place for you are considered. All these things can help you drive forward towards success. Do you need a computer? Is it up to date? Do you need Wi-Fi? Will it connect? If little things like this cause problems, then get a better environment or fix it and fix it quickly. Don't waste time on it. Cover all your bases. Make sure nothing will stand in your way and you have a back-up plan to take down any issues. If you have a list and you have all the barriers and what you can do to work around them, have your fail-safe in place. If something new comes up, then get it down and find a solution. Don't have problems anymore, create solutions. Be the person that solves all the issues and then when you do get it written down in the notepad, you know how to beat those problems time and time again until it becomes routine and you are always winning. Be that person; the person to turn too to solve all the problems. You will become more valuable and get further ahead. But most importantly, don't be that person for others. Be that person for you, your family, your friends, and the people that are important to you. Make your life better and the life of your family better by being the person that overcomes the barriers and sorts out the problems, especially your own.

Be independent. Learn everything you need to know about the best life for you and for what you want. Speak a little less and watch and listen a little more, as you will learn more this way. You can see and hear a lot more than you will ever learn from talking. Talk at the right time and do so for you to learn about you and how you can improve for yourself, and in turn, be a better you for you and your family. Take time and let the pace of life go a bit slower, so you can enjoy it and see the potential and the opportunity out there. There is so much opportunity out there and taking action at the right time can help you to move forward and get what you want or what you need. Most importantly, the life you want or the enjoyment in life you want. Even bad things that happen to you are a great opportunity–a chance to change direction and still move forward. You just need to see past the bad things and see how you can get a great benefit from the situation.

Chapter 3-Health: Diet, Exercise, and Sleep

I came across health, fitness, and diet about 20 years ago. In my last few years in school, I can remember a friend of mine was into it and I followed suit. I joined a gym at about 16 and it has always been something I have enjoyed, well most of the time, anyway. I can remember a few times when I have hated it. I ended up making it a big part of my career. I worked in a gym and I have gone on to train others to work in gyms. I still have a passion for it to this day and the nutrition side of it fits in quite naturally once you get into it. When it comes to sleep, I have never been much of an expert apart from the fact I am really good at it and I can't remember ever really having a bad night's sleep. I have read a book or two on the subject and it has helped me slightly. I owe a lot to the fitness industry. It has given me a great career which I really enjoy and couldn't see myself doing much else.

Let's start with a bit about diet. First and foremost, everyone wants a good diet, but they don't want to eat food that they don't like the taste of or that takes a long time to make. I could write a whole other book on this subject, as I have worked in that industry for quite a few years and have learned quite a lot about it. I may even do so; I have a project I started working on years ago, which I may go back to at some point. To make sure your diet is balanced, there are some fundamental guidelines out there with the general message; it is to portion your diet with a percentage from fruit and vegetables, a percentage from grains and carbohydrates, a percentage from fats, dairy, meats and minimal from sugars. By the way, you do need carbohydrates despite what some diet books say. The guidance is around 50% of your diet, although it does vary depending on different factors and I would say that is a little high. The main thing is to not shy away from the grains. It's more of the high-fat foods such as cakes, biscuits, doughnuts etc. that can cause a problem. They advise protein, but you don't need a high amount; normally around 15% again. This doesn't have to be exact and can come from a range of sources, such as milk, yogurt, cheese, eggs, nuts, lentils, chickpeas, and most meat. I would advise against supplementation unless you can't eat most of these foods listed due to dietary requirements, allergies, etc. Fats are normally guided at about 30% with it being mainly good fats from things like avocado, fish, nuts, etc. Not the high-fat calorie-dense fats such as pizza, chips, burgers, etc. Keeping it basic. You know what food is good and you know what food is bad. The trick is to find good food you like and is easy to prepare without being time-consuming.

Consider doing food prep the night before if you work or don't have much time during the day. Everyone can find an extra ten minutes before bed to sort out some food for the next day. A good start is snack pots, a bit like what you may have for a toddler– small plastic tubs with chopped up snacks; a good four to five with different snack can really make a difference to your diet. I go with chopped carrots, cucumber, whole cherry tomatoes, cheese cubes, and grapes. You could also have nuts, but they can be high calorie or even different fruits such as strawberries, raspberries etc. I go with whichever is cheapest in the supermarket, as this probably means they are in season and from this country, whereas the expensive fruits are probably out of season and imported.

You should be consuming the right number of calories for you to maintain, sustain your weight, or increase/decrease, depending on your goal. You can control how much you weigh just by eating the right number of calories. If you overeat, then you will gain weight. If your calories are the right amount, you will stay the same, and if your calories are under, then you will lose weight. If you overeat by five calories a day, that's 35 calories a week, 140 a month, and your weight will gradually increase over time. That's how easy it is to gain weight, and most people don't know how many calories they should be consuming. You can work out how many you should consume by taking your body weight in kilograms and multiplying it by 25. So, for example, if I weigh 90 kg and multiply it by 25, that equals 2,250, which is the base metabolic rate (minimum number of calories needed if you do nothing all day, such as just lay in bed). You then add a percentage based on how active you are; so, 25% if you're not active (no exercise and a desk job), 50% for moderately active (exercise three days a week), and 100% for highly active (exercise six to seven days a week or five and an active job). So, 100% would be double to 4,500. That sounds a lot but if you were on that and wanted to lose weight, then you would decrease by 100-200 calories per day and then after 1-2 weeks if you were not losing weight, then you would decrease by another 100 calories and keep following the same pattern until it drops. When it drops, maintain that amount until it stops, then decrease again. I would advise recalculating once in a while if your weight drops, as that can affect your calories needed. Never drop below 1,200 calories per day, as it would not be safe. Once you get to your ideal weight, you can maintain the amount you are on. If you are ever in doubt, follow the fundamental guidelines or seek professional advice. The more you weigh, the more you need and the less you weigh, the less you need. I think the UK government recommends for an average man, 2,500 calories and for a woman, 2,000 calories. Use this as a guide. Remember, you want a balance. One of the easiest ways to monitor it is to write it down on paper or a notebook of what you are eating. Most packets have calories on them. Be careful with the weight of the item and the amount you consume, as packets can list per 100 grams and not always by the packet size. So, you may be consuming 500 grams and it could list 1/5 of that, so then times it by five.

Record everything that goes into your mouth, including drinks. A lot of people gain weight just from drink alone, whether it's alcohol or juice, milk, etc. Also, make sure you are getting the correct vitamins and minerals in your diet. Drink plenty of water. Three to four pints a day is a good amount. Maybe have a multi-vitamin tablet if you are not getting them all in through your diet. Those two simple things alone can make a massive difference to your health. You don't even need expensive vitamins and can stick to tap water. Maybe even add squash if you have to. Keep alcohol and caffeine down along with high-fat foods. All these things will affect how you feel and your mood alongside your weight and even your happiness. If you're recording your diet and calories, maybe even add how you feel with a face–smiley, sad or normal, etc. This can help to identify patterns of how the foods make you feel or how you feel when you choose certain foods. Having a coffee might make you feel good, but how are you feeling four hours later, and the same with high-fat, high-sugar foods. All of this should give you a knock-on effect on your health if you are eating right. Then you should feel good, feel fresh, feel healthy. This could do more than reduce your waistline. It could help with the reduced risk of illness such as high blood pressure and type 2 diabetes. It could also make you feel more confident in yourself. You might be more likely to go out and join a gym and meet new people. You might feel more confident with people and relationships. You might have more motivation to get out and do things and see people and hopefully, it will help contribute to your happiness. You may face peer pressure of people asking you to go out for a drink or something to eat. You can still make a choice from the menu that you know will be better for you. They may moan at you about it and even criticise. At the end of the day, it should be your choice. I wouldn't worry what people think because when you're in great shape and they are not, then they won't be criticising. Or they will, and it will just be down to envy, which is what it is half the time, anyway. Because they don't have the willpower that you do. Are you stuck in a habit or routine from childhood? Can you look at it and think, why am I consuming this? Is it because my parents gave it to me, and I like it, so I carried on eating it? You can make a choice rather than stay in this fixed routine with nothing ever-changing. Because remember, if you change nothing, then nothing will change. You can take full control of not just your diet, but your whole life. What is working well? What isn't working well? The past and the future don't matter, just now. Where are you right now and what can you do right now?

When you go to the supermarket, whatever you buy is what you are eating. If it's junk food, then you're eating it. So, maybe plan out your shop, create a list and stick to it. Don't get roped into the offers and all the junk food they are trying to push on you. Make your own choices rather than being sold what you didn't plan to buy. Plan out your meals by looking up recipes. Make them work for you. Are you short on time? Find ones that can be made quickly. Are you short on money? Find ones that are cheap or have few ingredients or something you can batch cook and freeze for weeks to come. Plan it out. Create a list and shop with it. Habits may take time to change, and if you don't want to, then you don't have to; it's your life. Plan it out to suit you. But if you don't try, then you won't succeed. Greatness awaits you. When you make changes, then everything will change for you. Face it head-on, tackle it, and embrace it. Your fears will not be realised. Fears hold everyone back and they are just thought to protect you, but you don't need protecting. Take control of your mind and don't let it stop you.

Easy calorie reductions could be swapping foods such as crisps for popcorn, changing take away burger choice to a different one that has a lot fewer calories than others. Taking soda drinks out of your diet would remove a lot of calories. Coffees, lattes, and cappuccinos carry a lot of calories compared to black or black with milk. Alcohol carries a load of calories. Look at options with less if you can't cut it out, such as vodka or gin with a diet mixer. But I would advise of getting rid of it completely to help you find ultimate health. Plan healthy, think healthy, eat healthily, be healthy. Get yourself a calorie counting app if it helps and log everything you eat for a day, a few days, or even a week. You may be surprised by how many calories you are eating. Whatever you do, log it somehow, and get an idea of what you are eating and what you are putting in your body. Eat and drink for you, for life, and for health. Stop doing it for the taste. You can give yourself something once a day for the taste that isn't a high-calorie food choice. You're not a child anymore. You're a person that can make their own choices and make the right choices. You're someone that can take control of your life and be you without having to follow a crowd and without being influenced. You can be the person that leads the crowd and you can be the person that influences other people. You can be the one eating healthy food that tastes good and isn't a load of processed rubbish. Live a better life for you because eating better food will make you feel so much better, so much healthier, and you will look better. You may even have a better complexion and some colour in your skin. Break the cycle, break the routine, buy different food this week. Buy a completely different shopping trolley of food from what you normally do. Have the best looking, healthiest looking trolley in the supermarket. Be proud to push that trolley around. Don't be ashamed of it. Look at everyone else's and feel sorrowful for them, feel pity for them as they haven't taken control as you have. Swap out your coffee and tea for caffeine-free alternatives that will bring with it great health benefits, such as mint or chamomile tea. Keep hydrated, let other people complain and moan at you. If they do, then you know you're winning. You know you're doing the right thing as people hate others' success. So, use that to fuel your determination. Use it to fuel your fire to keep moving forward. Smile at them and ask them if they would like to try it, join you, or even if they would like to be a bit healthier.

With exercise, decide what is right for you, what fits with you, what works for you. Now, there is the recommended guidelines of about 30-60 minutes of moderate exercise a day, 3-5 days a week, and daily stretching. But you must do what fits you. Something is better than nothing if you can't hit the guidelines. Ideally, if you are going to the gym, then aim for 3-4 days a week, as a good level to see progress. The more you do, the faster you will get results. It's that simple. Anything you can do will help, including health and lifestyle changes. We have covered diet but think about things like walking more, using the stairs if you are a lift user, all the basics you might have heard people talk about. Vacuum more, remember a cleaner house equals an improved state of mind.

What sort of exercise should you do? So, do a warm-up, cardio for at least five minutes, but build it up a good 10-30 minutes a day. Three to four days a week at a moderate level will help. But even five minutes will help you to build up your fitness over time. Remember, slow and steady wins the race—the tortoise and the hare. A steady pace week in week out would be better than a few hard sessions and giving up because it's too much. Start off light and build it up. Rome wasn't built in a day. Daily stretching and core at home for 10 minutes. No need to leave the house; no gym needed. Check out basic exercises on YouTube or online, join a gym and get the advice of a trainer or maybe even a free session and a free plan. If you don't want to stay, ask them for a workout that you can do at home. With weight-based training, aim to do it three days a week, minimum, or even one day a week, and build it up. Even the social aspect of working out can help. Get in there and enjoy it; nothing else matters. It will all come in time. Try beginner's gym-based exercises, full-body workout covering the major muscle groups. You could do that in as little as two exercises. You could do deadlift and press-ups, not really beginner exercises, but just to give you an idea of how little you can do to fully work your body. You could do a 20 minutes weight work out and get in and out in no time; well 20 minutes. Then ideally, a good five to eight exercises as a beginner is a good amount if you can fit it into your day.

Speak to a trainer, tell them how much time you have, and get them to design a session based around that. You might not even have to pay for it. That could come back to your balance chart. Do you have spare money? Is your health low or vice versa; that should help you decide. Remember to finish with a cool down and a stretch off, drink plenty of fluid, wear suitable gym attire, and most of all, make sure you enjoy it. You can talk to people and socialise. If you enjoy it, then you will be more than likely to go back. If you don't want to talk to people, then maybe listen to music. If that's what you enjoy, remember this is part of your day, your time, and you should be making the most of it. Maybe even have a set playlist, not just for the gym; one for making you feel good, one for relaxing, and even one for the car. In the gym, make sure you have the correct technique and you are doing everything safely. See a trainer if you are not sure. You don't really need supplementation if you have your diet right. We covered vitamins and hydration earlier. If you have that in place, then you should be fine. Key point - protein powder is more processed than a Big Mac.

A basic weights workout would have legs, back, chest, shoulders, core and even some arm work. For cardio, you could use a range of the equipment including treadmill, bike, rower, cross trainer or stepper. You don't have to use all of them. You may just want to use one. Start with a warm-up, say five minutes walking. Cardio aims for 10-30 minutes at a moderate level, so on a scale of 1-10, if you were going to judge it on how hard it is, then 10 will be the hardest. You would work at about a six to eight level. Your heart rate when you would workout should be at about 70-80% of your maximum heart rate, which is worked out by taking your age away from 220. So, if you were 20 years old, take that away from 220 you get 200, which is your max heart rate. Then you would take away 20-30% to get the left-over heart rate level for your 70-80%.

For weight-based training, you would work about 10-15 reps, working so you feel it at the end, but not too hard that you can't do it. You should also have intervals of two to three times with a rest of about 30-60 seconds and a controlled tempo of two seconds each way. Remember, this is for a beginner and you will come across plenty of different training approaches. They can be varied later, but just use it as a starting point. You may feel sore or stiff the next day; the stretching should help limit that. Hopefully, you will see the benefits and they will come quicker the more days you do. Respect other people and be nice and civilised. You may even make new friends.

There is a range of different places you can train, including leisure centres, gyms, sports centres, cross-fit, or even clubs, including running, squash, tennis, etc. You can do memberships, even pay as you go, or some may even do trials/free periods. Remember, it's about you and what you want to do and there's no set way to it. Take it head-on and do what you will enjoy the most and provide you with the best results. You could even go to exercise classes, which proved a range of different options, including the classics such as circuits, Pilates, yoga, and aerobics. You also have a lot of new ones which are always changing depending on the current trends. Most places have a timetable, and these can be more motivating because you have an instructor, and they can be more social because there's a group of people.

You could always do a sport such as swimming or running, or even a team sport, or just going for a daily walk. If you don't enjoy it, then it won't work because you will probably give up. So, find something you like. Think about what you have done previously, what you have enjoyed, what you haven't enjoyed, and what you have done in school. What sports do you like or dislike? Even if you just get a bike and go cycling or go to the gym and just use the bike and nothing else, or even the rower or join a rowing club, there are a lot of options out there. It's about finding what works for you. Not everyone enjoys it and most people don't at first, which is fine. If you can maintain a moderate level, that's a good start, because once you start seeing results or when it gets easier, then it becomes more enjoyable. You will feel fitter, feel better, and that alone can keep you going. If you have it as a part of your plans or goals, then you could make smart goals around it and short, medium and long-term goals. These can be laid out from a health or fitness perspective. So, you might want to lose so much weight by a set time and measure it with scales and do it through exercise and diet. Get it all down on paper and know exactly how what why and when.

If you know someone that goes (a friend or family member), then you could join them, or you might want to go to get away from them as you may have that quite high on your lifecycle as it is and you may need time to yourself. This could cover multiple parts of your cycle, health, spending time with family, and saving money, as you have a membership at the gym, and it takes you away from spending it on doing other things. It's worth considering. At the very least, try and get more active or increase or progress what you're doing gradually. Don't overdo it. Do what your body can cope with and make sure you get that balance with rest. Move forward but ride the wave. You may be paddling forward in the water against the waves, but every now and again, a wave will come along that you will want to ride. So, take it and ride it. Just be careful you don't fall off. When you walk in a gym, if you walk in a gym, there may be that moment of anxiety, that moment where you fear everyone is looking at you, that you feel people may be judging you. Well, they aren't. They are thinking the same thing you are unless they have been there a while, and they have forgotten about it. They are just in another place, like a supermarket or pub, just without the food and drinks. Instead, it's protein bars, bananas, and shaker bottles. That time will come if you do, by some random chance, get someone staring at you. Then put it down to jealousy or something else; insecurities, maybe. That's what most of them are about and that's why most are in the gym in the first place. We all want to work on something and improve something. We're all striving for the impossible of perfection, thinking we might achieve it. Because if we didn't think it, then nothing would really motivate us to do something about it. Or, I guess they may just fancy you. If we allow this fear to conquer us, we would all become motionless, with no desire or passion to get anywhere. So, get in the gym, be the person judging everyone else, and do it for entertainment value, as you get all sorts of characters in the gym. The more muscular and prettier they are, then the friendlier or more insecure they are. Get training, get moving, and get your body in better shape. No one will do it for you, and it won't happen next year. It has to happen now. Keep going until it's a habit and you enjoy it. Then after that, it will become easy.

How important is it that you exercise? Well, it depends how you feel about yourself, it depends how much you get out of the house and do something, it depends on how good your diet is, and on how active you are in life, and other areas. If you are in good shape, you feel good about yourself, you have a clean diet, and you are active, then you may not need it that much. If you tick some of these, then it may help you. If you tick none of these, then I would get down to the gym now and sign up.

Do you have a social life? Are you depressed? Would it do you good to be around people? Then go, go, go, and once you have signed up, then get booked into some of the classes and meet new people. Most of them are there for the same reason. Remember, even in the class, don't go too hard to begin with. Build it up slowly. Try out different classes, try out different training programmes in the gym, make sure you rest for a week after every four to six weeks of training, and then when you go back, try something different–a different programme, a different class, vary depending all of this and depending on your goal. Change your goal to give you variety, don't just have one. Have two or three and make them relevant to you, your purpose, your values, and make them smart and achievable. Make sure you plan them over time. Go back to the chapter about planning and goal setting if you need to. Speak to a trainer in the gym if it helps. Don't take their response as an answer, though. Speak to more than one trainer and try to gauge if you are getting an opinion or something true to their training. These guys can tend to go off script and start spouting beliefs over true knowledge of key principles of training and exercise. Even do some further research yourself if you need it. Make sure you research it from a reputable source. There is so much garbage online, so be careful with it. You can't go wrong if you just put in the training, day after day, and leave feeling like you have worked out. If you leave feeling great, then you probably haven't worked hard enough. Don't kill yourself, but make sure you're puffing a little bit, sweating a little bit, and then cool down before hitting the showers and heading home for some rest.

How can we incorporate sleep into our balance with a good amount and with good quality sleep? So, how much sleep is needed? I believe the guidance is eight hours. You could go either side of this, say with 7 ½ to 8 ½, but the key thing is what is right for you. Is the amount you're having now making you feel more tired? Is it making you feel drowsy? It could be worth experimenting with different amounts of times and with different times of going to bed and getting up. Too much can be just as bad as not enough, sometimes with it making you feel tired and wanting more sleep. A good rest is the main thing. Don't worry too much about actually sleeping, just lie down and rest with your eyes closed. You will find that sleep will naturally come when it's ready or the key thing is to only go to bed when you are actually tired. Check the time, set your alarm for seven to eight hours later, providing it fits in with the time you need to get up for work or anything else planned.

Consider your sleeping environment. Is it clean, vacuumed, or do you have clothing on the floor? Is it messy? Do you have the right balance of light? What is the decoration like, or the wattage of your bulbs? Do you have plants in your room? Is your clothing folded up and tidy? Do you have a television on? Do you have your phone on? All these things can affect you, your sleep, and your ability to relax. Do you allow pets in your room? What's your bedding like–the pillows, the filling, the case material? Is it cotton or polyester? How old are they? Are they thin? How is your mattress? How old is it? How are the springs? Have you had it more than eight years? Do you have or need a mattress topper? Would you be better with Egyptian cotton sheets with a high thread count? What size is your bed? Is it the right size for you and the room? How thick is your duvet? Is it the right thickness for the time of year? How hard is your mattress or is it soft? Does your partner affect your space in bed or your sleep? What is the temperature of your room? Do you even know? Do you have the windows open? Do you have the thermostat set to a certain temperature? Do you lay on your back, front or side? Which side? Maybe consider which gives you the best night's sleep; try out different things. I believe if you are right-handed, then it is recommended to sleep on your left side and vice versa. I may be wrong about that.

Consider your routine. The hour before, are you having a bath or a shower like you might have done when you were a kid? Have you shut off from work? When did you last eat? Was it within the last hour? What is your mindset? Take control of your mindset in every aspect of your day. If you are in traffic, and it's upsetting you or stressing, you take control of yourself and realise you are not going to end up on a beach in a hot country by getting angry. So, get a grip and just relax and enjoy your day and the moment. Keep your emotions in check and take control because once you do, you will be happier and get more out of your day so that you can wind down at the end of the day. Don't get so wound up that you must wind down that much. Remember, you could have a bath before bed, then maybe even do 10 minutes of yoga or 10 minutes of meditation or even both. You could work on breathing exercises as part of it. You could have a journal from your day, writing down what you have achieved from the day, what has been a success. You could layout your goals for the following day. What you want to achieve, including your to-do list and your dreams, from the previous chapter. This can help clear your head, but it can also make you feel good from what you have achieved in the day. This can also help clear your mind. You have the next day planned out, which can prevent you from forgetting anything or worrying about anything–appointments, things to pick up, drop off, stuff you must do.

How do pets affect your sleep? Do they jump on the bed, or scratch at the door if you don't let them in the room, barking or meowing? Have they been fed? Is it best to put them out for the night or give them their own space/room? How about partners needing a hug, which could affect the temperature or space? Do they want attention, want to talk, or something else? Do you need to go to bed an hour earlier to spend time with them or whatever time you need? Would this maybe even help you to relax? Could it help your relationship and bonding, considering another part of the lifecycle? Power naps could be taken during the day, which could also help with your overall wellness; maybe around midday to early afternoon. Try to avoid going past 2 o'clock, as it could affect you later when it comes to sleeping. It can help make you feel fresh for the rest of the day. Time is important, as too much can make you feel worse. So, the optimum time is about 20-30 minutes. Much more than 30 minutes can make you sluggish and tired, so maybe set an alarm for about 25 minutes after you lay down. So, you may be at work. How do you do this? Well, you have a break, is it 30 minutes? Go to your car. If you have to, eat for 10 minutes, put the heating on, and find a mellow radio station. Maybe lock your car for safety. Remember, you don't have to sleep, just relax, and if you do fall asleep, then bonus. Make sure your engine is turned off. Make sure you are in a quiet location with not many people walking by.

Consider your clothing in bed, not for your power nap; although you may want a blanket and a travel pillow if you want to go all out. But in bed, you may wear underwear, pyjamas, whatever you feel comfortable in. Make the most of everything thing out there that can give you the best sleep possible. Don't let up on it. Use everything in your power to make it the best possible sleep and sleeping environment.

What are the answers to all these questions I have just asked? Well, only you should really know that because it is what works for you and what helps you to have the best night's sleep. What I want you to do is to be aware of all these different things, not when going to bed but in theory of planning the best night's sleep for you and testing and trying out different ways to see if they help you or not. But don't let it bother you; just try bits out. If you are already comfortable sleeping, well then you may not need any of them or you may be able to identify the odd thing that might make it even better and even more comfortable. You deserve to have a clean, comfortable sleeping environment with a room fit for a king or queen, even if it's with a single bed.

Sleep deprivation is the worst kind of torture, so get this right, as you don't want to live a life of torture; you want the opposite. So, get some good sleep. Try these things out; implement new bits at a time. You don't have to do everything at once. You may be lucky enough to be able to sleep 4 or 5 hours a night and feel great the next day. Our bodies can adapt and can adapt well. If you must start getting up at five every morning, then eventually you would be able to do it without an alarm clock, as you would adapt to it.

Do your kids disrupt your sleep? Have they got a good sleeping environment? Have they drunk too much before bed? Have they had a good wind-down routine? Have they had too much sugar late in the day? Get their sleep to the level you want your sleep to be and then you can all sleep well, with a better life, with less stress, and a lot more recovery time. Your bedroom should be an environment that you love going into. If you are spending eight hours a night sleeping in there, then that is one-third of your day; 33.3% of your day is in that room, maybe more. So, make it a great room and make it a great place that you look forward to being in. This can then be the same for other environments–your car, your workplace, your kitchen, your front room, wherever you spend the most time, depending on your situation. These things alone make life a little bit better, more enjoyable, and easier to deal with; and we all know life isn't that easy to deal with. At least get this part right. At least get it together with this key element to your health. Then the other bits can come as and when if you really want them. This can just look after you, your body, your mindset, and your mental health, which is more important than anything. Because without your brain, you won't operate. So, look after it. If you lose it, then you lose everything.

Chapter 4–Your Home, Environment and Ambience, Leisure, Travel, and Media

Over the years, I have come to learn from living with a range of different people that a clean and tidy living space is highly important to you, being happy. No one wants to live in a dirty, messy place where you can't find anything. I have struggled to live with people that chuck stuff on the floor and don't tidy up after themselves. I make as much effort as I can to not live like that–to keep belongings to a minimum, and to make sure everything has a place. That way, it is easy to find and stress free, with a nice living environment that I can enjoy living in. I have also learnt to take this forward to my travel space (car) and to make sure it works for me and is somewhere that I like being rather than just another place. If you make every room in your house and your car somewhere that you are happy to be in and like being, then your life will be a little bit better.

This will cover areas such as where you live, your surroundings, the layout, the design, the colour of the paint on the walls, the lighting, the mood, the sounds and how it all affects you, your mindset and your emotions; which could affect you and the way you are and your behaviour. Look at chickens and hens and how they are kept, with some in cages and some which are free range. How does it affect their mood, health, and wellbeing? How do you live compared to this? Do you go out much? Do you enjoy what you have around you? How happy are you? What is your balance like on this topic? How tidy is your house? Do you put things away or is it chucked in a cupboard or just chucked anywhere? Do you keep the place tidy? Where do you keep your clothing? Is it in drawers and folded or is it left out in a heap?

Where do you put your work stuff? Is it left out and calling you back to check emails, etc. or do you shut it down and put it away? Where do you keep your keys? Do you struggle to find them or are they kept in an easy to find a place where they can be found? It can be less stressful if you know where everything is and can find them with ease. Do you make your bed in the morning or do you leave it and come home to a mess?

What's the lighting like? Do you have enough? Is it bright enough? Do you have a dimmer? Do you have suitable wattage for the size of the room? Do you have something you can play music on? What music do you have? Do you have music that can help you get ready for your day and music that you can put on at the end of the day to help you relax? Consider the layout and what best suits your needs. Cover all the basics–make it a clean, presentable, nice place to be–then you will be happier from that alone. It makes it easy for you to be happy, or do you want to make it hard to be happy? Where do you eat your food? At the table, on the sofa, in your room? Does this make areas smelly or messy? Keep everything clean, the bedsheets, your clothing, the carpets; it will all help.

How many plants do you have? Aim for at least one per room, maybe even two? Go for easy to maintain plants that don't need much watering and can survive with limited light. They don't just make the rooms look nice, they can help clear the air, removing toxins. Do you have photos up of family to make it feel more homely? Do you have mirrors up? Again, aim for one in every room, opposite to windows, they can help reflect light in.

What colours are your carpets and walls? Are they bright? Do they need a new coat of paint? Are they fresh-looking? Does your furniture suit your house and make you feel comfortable? Does it suit your style and your values? Try to appreciate and look after everything you have. Value it and take care of it. It will last longer and make you happier, as you won't need other things because you will have everything you need. Be grateful for the small things, like a roof over your head, a bed to sleep in, a fridge with food in it. Some people don't have these things. So, if you do, then look after them, make them look like new. Gratitude brings happiness. Make sure all rooms are clean, the bathroom, for example, don't have things out all over the side. Have a place for them. Make each room somewhere you want to go; somewhere you want to spend time.

Do you need everything you have? Can you throw things out, sell them online, or even donate them to charity? Do you have old clothing you don't wear? Could you give it to someone who needs it? How is your garden? Do you have plants? Do you cut the grass regularly? Are your plants easy to maintain? Does it look fresh? Ask the question, is this somewhere I want to be? If not, then make it somewhere you want to be; make it somewhere everyone wants to be. How about your car; how clean is it? Do you like it? Does it feel dirty? Can you make it spotless, inside and out? Look at the same model for sale online, the same age from a trade seller and see how clean it is. Can you make yours look like that? How much better do you feel when it's clean? Clear out anything you don't need. You may need a jack, water, high vis jacket, etc., but you can clear out a lot of the stuff you don't need. A vacuum can make most places look a lot nicer. Consider an air freshener, not just for the car but your home. A nice smelling environment is always good. Once you get all this in place, maybe have a schedule in place to keep on top of it. You shouldn't have to be doing it all the time, but you should want to keep on top of it. Do you have spare money? Can you pay someone to clean your house once a week to save time? Which is more valuable to you? Which do you need to work on within your cycle?

Do you take care of yourself? Are you clean? Do you wash daily? Do you keep everything trimmed? Do you moisturise? Do you try to be presentable with your clothing? Do you make every effort to make yourself look good? Are you covering the exercise element? Are you doing core exercises and yoga, etc.? Do you feel like a million bucks when you get dressed? You should. You should feel great every day with what you wear. All this can contribute to your mindset and how you feel. How are your emotions? Ultimately, are you happy and do these things affect you? We will touch more on this in the happiness section, but the book should bring all this together to get you in a good place. People won't even have to ask. They will see you are good, and they will get this from your body language alone.

Do you sit straight? Are your shoulders back, or are they dropping? Do you walk with a spring in your step or drag your heels? Switch it up; show people you are great. Bring it all together, let people know without even talking. Compare it to a plant that hasn't been watered for a week, drooping, struggling to live. Give it water and it will change in no time to being upright and radiant with life. Is this what is affecting you? How much water do you drink? Have you had three pints for the day or have you had none for weeks because all you drink is coffee?

Do you let things affect you? Do you have control over your mindset? Do you do things at the right time? It's true what they say. Timing can be everything. That's why sometimes people put things off. They are waiting for the right time, for it to feel right, for them to be in the right emotional state, or for the person they are talking to be in the right frame of mind. If you are not in the right mindset, then it could be best to wait, take control and be honest with people if you don't want to talk about it. Think about the film "Yes man." The protagonist says yes to everything, and it changes his life. I wouldn't recommend it, but maybe, to some degree, loosen up and be more flexible. Say yes first, then work it out. Don't say no, then shut down. Don't say yes to stuff you don't want to do or stuff that is illegal, but be more positive and then life will be more positive for you. You can even tell from someone's tone of voice, more so than the words they say. Take control of this. You can say whatever you want if you do it in the right tone and with the right body language and get away with it.

The only person that can bring sadness to you is yourself. I think Nelson Mandela when asked about being in prison once said, "They can take your body, but they can't take your heart and your mind." Which shows clearly that you can be in a bad place and still have control over your happiness and self without letting others win or beat you down. There will be a lot of ups and downs in life, good and bad. But never dwell on the ups or the downs. Enjoy the highs, but don't let the lows beat you, even though they will always fire back up. Sometimes when you are at the lowest point, you have no way to go but up.

The other thing to remember is that nothing is permanent; everything is temporary. Everything that is born will die, including the planet. Everything will come to an end. You may still exist in the form of your remaining molecules as everything goes back to that form and changes; everything changes form at some point. Anything bad that happens, learn from it. If you fail at something, then learn from it. That didn't work. How else can you approach it? Learn from how you fail. Attack it a different way; there's more than one way to skin a rabbit. If you don't succeed, then try again. Only you can do it, and if you don't, then nothing will come of it.

What will it take? What will make where you live perfect for you? What will make it clean and fresh? You might be okay with it being a mess, as it may save you time by not cleaning it. The point is, what will make it right for you? How would you like it to be for you? How could it be better? That is the question, and if I could ask you the same questions, again and again throughout this book, then it would be: how would you like life to be for you? How could it be better? What would make life comfortable for you, and how would you like it to be? There is not a book on this planet that has your answer, as the answer is in you. It may help to read books to help generate your thinking or you may get ideas or learn something new, but most of the answers to your questions are within you.

Let's start with travel. Travel time can be consuming, it can take up a big part of your life and I know that more than most people. If its work travel, holiday travel, or whatever, you don't want to waste that time; make the most of it, make that environment perfect for you, make it comfortable, enjoyable, and be grateful for it. What's your car condition? Is the seat right for you? Is the car right for you? Do you have air in the tyres? Are the fluid bottles topped up? Is it clean? Have you vacuumed it? Are the pockets clear of rubbish? Is the glove box clear of rubbish? Do you have emergency supplies–food, water, first aid kit, sweets in the glove box for when you are in traffic jams? A blanket in case you want a power nap. Do you have a spare jacket for if you break down to keep you warm on the side of the road? Do you have a suitable spare tyre? Do you have enough fuel for your journey? Do you have everything you need? What about comfortable clothing, shoes, etc.? Planning out your journey, including time and stops, saves you rushing, then you can be sure that you can stick to the speed limit and be on time; no stress of worrying about being pulled over. It's fine even if you are going to be late because you will want to make it to your destination. Let people fly by you, watch them, and be prepared to get out of their way or stop. Because that should be your focus, not avoiding getting a ticket or being pulled over. Consider planning comfort, accessories, anything you might need; maybe even a coffee flask. Even a travel pillow again for that nap, if needed. Maybe a playlist that you have created or audiobooks so you can learn while you are travelling, or even downloaded podcasts. Whatever works for you and makes it great for you, it shouldn't be average, it should be great, and you should be able to travel in comfort and make the most of your time.

Are you making the most of your leisure time? Are you resting enough? Have you slept enough? Are you getting a power nap in? Do you get everything done that you have planned to complete? Do you have a much-needed break when you need it, even if it's 10 minutes? Just switch off, be late home by 10 minutes if you must, be a bit fresher, get more done and have no issues at the end of the day. Take it away from work, in your car or go for a walk; somewhere away from where you spend most of your time. Shut that phone down and just enjoy the world for 10 minutes–no screens, no people that you already know; strangers are fine. Meet new people, walk in the local park or high street, go to a library or a different coffee shop than the usual. Breathe, focus on your breathing and feed your body what it needs–clear fresh oxygen. Maybe take a break when you get home. Don't just shut down and give up on the day, take a break, then get on with the things you want to do with your life. Own your time, own your life, and start moving forward. Don't let anything hold you back. If you can't afford a spa or a massage, go for a walk on the beach. Get away from the norm and do something different. Take some time off work and go on holiday. Find a new level of energy. Find a positive emotional mindset. Take control of your cycle and balancing it out and work on those low areas.

In terms of media, phones have it all. Use it, get the app–get the meditation apps, the yoga app, the podcasts, the audiobooks, and the music. Get everything you need to support your leisure and travel time and make sure you use them. Stop playing games on your phone and start making yourself healthy. There is no easy fix to this; it's like a drug, so go cold turkey. Delete, purge all those apps that consume your life and give you nothing back. Only have ones that give you something back or have a use–app for online banking, calorie counters, running mapping, education. Do you need news, social media and games? Okay, you might want some for leisure time, especially streaming videos, etc. But cap it; limit it. Should you be letting it consume you seven days a week? Imagine what you could achieve in life if you put your television time into something else or even your social media time. I bet you could learn a language in a year or set up a business to produce a second income. But it's up to you. What do you even want in life? Whatever it is, make sure you get it because if you didn't get it yesterday, you probably won't be getting it tomorrow. So, when? Make that plan and put it on top of your list, then break it down into days per week and hours per day. Then work out when you will achieve it; add the days up and you should be able to find your end date.

If you are down, unhappy, sad, or depressed, then it might take longer. Make yourself happy and you will smash it out the park. You will be there so much sooner. Yes, you can make yourself happy because you have control over your mind; so, do it. Focus on it and believe it. If you don't believe it, then it won't happen because your mind is always right, and it always makes things how you think they will be. But that's fine because it's possible to take control of your mind and shut out all the shit in life. Use everything in your power to get there. If you want to work on a goal after a long day at work, then, by all means, have a strong coffee and high-sugar foods if it helps. It won't help when you have the sugar crash, but it may help you for the moment that you want to reach your goals. So, abuse it, take advantage of it, use everything in your power to win and own your time. The key thing here is all of these things can really consume your time. Leisure well great if it helps you to recover. Get some downtime and come back fresh to work towards your mission and even greater if it brings you happiness and doesn't have a negative effect on other areas in your life, such as family.

Travel may not be avoidable as you may need it for work or depending on the location you live in. So, as per the key points in this section, make sure you make the most of that time. Media, television, online, socialising, and even games, especially games. All these things can really consume our time, and we let them. This really is a crossover into leisure, as some people use these as leisure-time activities. How much of our time do we let this consume is up to us? Do we plan it? Do we monitor it? Probably not. Do you think we should? We work to a fixed routine and time for work. Why can't we do it for our downtime? It's up to you. Do you think it will help you to plan other things into your time that you want to achieve and may not be achieving? Will it help you? Then maybe it is worth considering. It's your time. Do with it as you please. But if for one second you feel like it's being wasted, then it probably is being wasted. What do you want from your time and life? Do you need that downtime when you are watching television or while scrolling on your phone? Yes, you do. But how much time do you need to apply to that? That is probably the key question in this whole section, as it should get you thinking about your time and how you use it and what it means to you.

The other fundamental thing to take away is how you use your time when you have no control over it. Going back to the travel time, how can you make the most of it? That is the other key point to take away. Go back over if you need to and think beyond the book about what you can do for you and how you can put something into place that would benefit you and your life.

Chapter 5– Work and Money

I think I would be in good company if I was to say that there have been times in my life when I haven't wanted to work for a living. I guess most people feel that way at some point. I have managed to make it past that through finding work I enjoy, work that I wanted to do. It helped get me to a point where it doesn't really feel like work. If you can do that, find your dream job or something you would love doing, then you will get to a place where you will be going to work, but it won't feel like work. It's just something you like doing. I feel very lucky to be in this position and it did take me years of training and years of applying for jobs, but I got there eventually. I nearly gave up at one point and I am so glad I didn't.

I probably grew up like most in a low to medium income household. I don't ever really feel like I went without and I have great memories of my childhood. I can assure you of one thing though, and that is that my parents had a mindset of not overspending and not wasting money–turn the lights off, turn the tap off, the heating would rarely be on, and things would be bought at discounted prices and with vouchers, and so on. I have come to learn the last few years that even if you don't have much, that this is no way to live. It is only adding to your problem. If you are that thrifty, then you should look at ways of solving it rather than accepting it and living in such a way. That comes across a bit brutal, but it has really helped me. Trying to save every penny actually won't help much at all. It will just make you feel down as it adds to the feeling that you can't afford things when you can. You shouldn't have to live like that. I take nothing away from my parents. They worked hard and gave me everything I could have ever wanted, and I learnt from them how to work hard. I have them to thank for my persistent hard-working ethics and it has helped me to see that no one is perfect, and you can always change the way you live.

How you manage your time is everyone's favourite topic. Well, sleep can take up a third of your life, well sort of–eight hours work, eight hours sleep and eight hours for everything else; unless you modify the balance of time and sleep less and work more, or whatever you want to do with it. This also doesn't account for retirement if you make it that far. How do we get a good balance? How do we get happy with it? Well, it can be as simple as finding a job you like; some people never truly find what they want to do. So, write down your likes, what you enjoy doing, and what interests you. Do a bit of research on jobs that match those interests or jobs that you might like. It doesn't matter what age you are. Consider the suitability with the working hours, the pay, the location and everything else. Consider all your options and then get back to school. Research course options. You don't have to do a degree, but don't rule it out. Can you do something similar with a short course? Can you do an evening course? Can you learn on the job? Don't rule anything out. If it means doing a distance learning degree online for five years with limited support to achieve a dream job, then it might just be worth it. If you get the training and get the job you want, then life can become a lot easier and you can even end up in a job where you don't feel like you're working. I've done it myself. I worked jobs I haven't enjoyed, worked long hours. I have also retrained and made it into jobs I've always wanted to do, with a lot of hard work and attending evening courses or taking days off to attend training courses. What extra time can you find to attend a course? Maybe doing one in the evening. How much research have you done? Some people get home and watch television every night or sit on their phones for hours; they might watch a movie. Why not invest that time in something that will give you something back for it? What about looking at different career options/paths and different training options? You could take that one night a week to attend a training course or spending that time at home doing an online course. Can you afford it? Are there cheaper options? Can you get support from your government or bursaries? If you're in a job you don't like, then maybe even try to become great at it, as it will become a lot more enjoyable. You may become one of the best in your company rather than being one of the worst. You will feel a lot more content.

Are the people at work happy? Nope. Are they working hard? Maybe, but is it 100% effort? Unlikely? How much time do you put in? Do you work too much or not enough? Are you giving your employer value for money for what they pay you? Do you make yourself so valuable they can't afford to lose you and want to give you everything to stay? Do you utilise your time? Fit as much work into it as possible to free up time for you? The more you can get done in the shortest time, then the more time you will have. You can become time rich. Time is the thing we have so little of, but we waste so much of it. You trade your time for money so you will be better off as a whole. Think about how you utilise your time. Plan out your day. Do you have that to-do list in place? Can you get up earlier and knock through it? What is the best time for you to do it? Do you operate better at night or in the morning? What is your work environment like? Do you like it? Is it clean? Are you comfortable there? Is it a space in your home? Do you have a desk? Is it tidy? Do you have a great green plant on your desk? Do you drink coffee? Are you hydrated enough? How much water are you having? Are you buying coffee or taking your own? Would you save money by making your own? Think about the finance side of the life cycle. Do you have a decent coffee flask that will keep it warm long enough? Invest in the right one and it could save you money. You could spend money to save money. A £20 flask that saves you spending £2 a day on coffee is saving you £20 after 10 days. A 5-day working week, and you are saving £40 a month; that could be your gym membership. Do you buy your lunch? If you could take it, you can save £3 a day, which means you could save a lot if you prepared and took your lunch in for the week.

But which do you need to work on the most, time or money? Now, I know that isn't the best or even an amazing money tip, but it may help some people. If you want great guidance on money, then look into stock market investing and learn as much as you possibly can about it, and it may open your eyes to what can be achieved. How about emails? Do you have that balanced or are they coming non-stop? Have multiple groupings in your inbox. Have one for information, one for things to follow up on, or any topic you feel relevant. Then move the emails over to the relevant folder to help clear, save all that is relevant in the right folder, then purge or mass delete the rest. Make sure you have all the important ones you need in the right folders, and then zero that baby out. Bring It back to empty and feel great. Sit there and smile as you look at that empty inbox. For follow-up ones, you can even set reminders in your diary to follow up with on set dates and times. Same with your diary, clear out anything you don't need, only open it when needed. Same with your emails; don't have them open all day. Open them once a day at a set time every day and only answer them then. Then sign-out and come back tomorrow. Own your emails; don't let them own you. If anything is urgent, then people can call you. Emails are a non-urgent form of communication. If someone doesn't realise that, then it can be their problem, not yours. Make people aware they can call you if it's urgent. The same with work. Set times and work through it, then come back the next day. Some of these things will be job specific. You may not have to deal with emails, or you may not have the luxury of planning out your working time. Working with colleagues can be good or bad, depending on who you work with and what they are like. People can complain a lot and be negative. Try to get away from them. Be around the positive people, the ones which will make you feel better. The negative ones will bring you down and affect you if you let them. Be professional; don't cross boundaries. I know this can be hard. But it will make life a lot better at work. You can be sociable, but try to behave appropriately. It can really cause problems and make the work environment uncomfortable. Remember, it's you and your life. You can do what you want, and you want to enjoy it as much as possible. You might not care about those things and really you shouldn't care about anything. Happiness should overrule the lot. If something makes you happy, then go with it, but just be careful that it doesn't crash down and bring you sadness. Make sure you understand the risk and the issues that can come with it.

How is the location of your work and commute time? Is it long? Do you make the most of it? Do you listen to the radio, music, audiobooks or podcasts, which can be a good way to learn and get through a lot of material? You can learn about a range of different topics which could come back to help you with your development–be it with health, work, family, finance, etc. Consider making the most of this time and managing your time. You could even listen to a book in the gym. You don't even have to do it every day. You could balance this time, one day with a book, one day with music, one day with no headphones and being sociable and talking to others, be it in the gym or on a train to work. You could even balance out your travel. You might take the train, you might drive, you could car share another day. Get a balance and do different things. Do things that help you to face your fears and provide you with variety. Face all your fears and see what comes of it. Whatever you do, you will be a long time doing it, so make it fun and enjoy as much of it as you possibly can.

Give your life fun and enjoy every moment you possibly can. Regardless of your work and what you do, you should have free time at home, and if you want to change what you do for work, then use that free time to support the change. Even if you're setting up your own business, plan in so much time a week to spend on it and start doing it, as with no action you will get no results and with a lot of action or massive action then you will get results. It may not be the results you want, so look at it and see what works, make changes and adopt different approaches. If something is working, then keep doing it and do it more and more and don't stop. Work for you and work for your family. Even if you made a great success of work and generated a great income, even a passive one where you didn't have to work, you should still want to work as income is the best source of money you will ever get. It will keep coming as long as you work, which shows how valuable you are to your job role. Now, I know it may not be enough and it never is enough because the more you have, the more you will be able to find to do with it. Even if you have everything you want, then one of the most sensible things to do with your money is to invest it and so even then the more you have the more you will want to invest, as that money will keep making you wealthier and wealthier or richer and richer. However you want to look at it, one key thing to take from this is not to work for money as you can earn a lot from a terrible job. This could be eight hours a day, five days a week, for 45 years. Do you really want to do that to yourself? That is pure madness. Find something that you are happy doing. If you must do two jobs that you love and work an extra day a week, then it might just be worth it.

Consider everything I have covered, including the conditions. Make your work great, make your life great. If you have a partner, then they must be supportive of what you do and understand why you do it. If they are not, then is that someone that you want in your life? You should have people with you that are fully supportive of you and your dreams and what makes you happy. So surround yourself with these people.

Live to work, don't work to live.

Money. Why do we have it? What is it for? To trade for goods, services, etc.? Maybe even luxuries, pets, spend on the family? The list could be endless and so could your spending. You earn money, then it comes in; you spend it, then it goes out. Simple. Do you spend more than you earn, or do you earn more than you spend? Does it bring happiness? Has it ever brought you happiness? I guess the real question is, has it brought you long term or permanent happiness? If you don't have enough, will it make you unhappy? If so, will this be permanent or temporary? Can it stop you from doing the things you want to do? It can be free to go out for the day and enjoy yourself; it's up to you if it costs anything. You could spend thousands going on holiday and have a bad time. You could go for a walk for free on your local beach and it could turn out to be an amazing time. Does it cost too much to eat healthily? People say it does. Well, maybe from a time perspective, it will cost you time, but money, no. It's a lot cheaper to cook yourself and to cook fresh local food. You could cook a meal for as little as £1 or maybe even less. People don't want to cook for one person. Why? Cook enough for five people and freeze it. You will then have four meals that you can use for the next four days. Do this every day for a week and you will be able to eat for weeks without buying food. Do you save your money? Do you invest it? Do you diversify? I guess the first basic step is to save. Save as much as you can each month, every month. Do it as soon as you get paid and then cover everything else. Try to limit all the expenditures. Do you need all those monthly payments going out? Build up a safety net in your account-£100, £200, £1000; whatever you can afford. See it as zero. Once your account hits that number, then you are out of money for the month. Have it as an overdraft or a rainy-day fund. Aim to save 10% each month as a minimum. If you can do more, then great. Maybe even 20%. Get a savings account, one with the highest interest rate you can get. Have multiple accounts, as many as you need. One for your monthly expenditure, one for your savings, and maybe even one for your dreams. Save money into it for your dream goal—a car, a holiday trip, a house, whatever it is.

With stocks and shares, just don't risk it. You will be playing poker with the greatest poker players in the world; you don't stand a chance. Get financial advice or learn it inside out and upside down. If you must invest, go for something like the FTSE 100 or S&P 500, use a company with really low rates so you don't lose money on your investment, for example, the company Vanguard. With property investment, you could get 8% + returns. Again, know the subject inside out. At least read three books minimum on anything you want to invest in; learn something about it first. Get a three-bedroom house up North in the UK, rent out the three rooms separately, cover the expenses, and you might make some money. Work out the ROI (return on investment) there is no point even starting if you are not making a profit on your investment. Would you start writing a book without reading some books first on how to write a book? At the very least, watch some videos online?

Do you have debt? Do you have credit cards? Get rid of it, if you have a mortgage fine, or debt that is returning you money? Do you have extra hours free that you can work on an extra job to use towards your debt? Can you wipe off or lower the interest on your debt by switching it to another bank? If working, get a pension plan. If your employer matches it, then it's a good deal. You will lose a bit based on it dropping, but that will be more than covered if your employer matches what you put in, which in theory doubles your money. But don't put it all in. It's like the old saying, "Don't put all your eggs in one basket." If you can have savings, pension, investments, and your dream account and build them up in that order, then you will be nicely spread out with your money and at a low risk of losing it all. If you can protect your income too, then even better if it has some sort of income insurance. Because if you lose your income, then you could be in trouble. It depends on how confident you are of replacing your job. Do you have kids? Do you want to save some for them for when they are older? Maybe ten pounds a week until they are 21 would build up a nice amount for their 21st birthday. Aim to keep that spending down, less than what you earn. Set a direct debit for your savings make it automatic.

How can you spend less? What is your weekly shop like? Do you waste money? Do you throw food away at the end of the week? Do you buy the most expensive option when you could buy cheaper? Can you reduce the payments going out of your account? Are there cheaper options? Can some be cancelled because they are not even being used? Can you then add that amount to your savings direct debit? In other words, pay yourself, give yourself a pay rise? Stop giving it to other people.

You work for it and one day might want it. Make it worth going to work, to earn money that you will keep for you that you might need for security or even an investment. Make your money work for you.

Keep investing. Use your money to earn you money because that is what money does best, earn money. You just have to learn where to invest it and what will provide you with the best return on investment. Don't worry about having debt if it makes money. If you buy a house with debt and rent it out and the rent covers your debt, then you're in theory getting a free house. Maybe even more if there is money left over after expenses. Save for your kids and yourself. Invest in yourself, spend on your education even if it's just reading books. Learn more about everything. Spend money wisely on your food. Junk food will not do you any good. You don't need coffee. Save all that money and see how you feel after a month. Junk food and coffee is the new cigarette. They cost money and do us no good. Get a spreadsheet in place, put all your expenditures on it. Log in to your online banking and look at the last month, record it, compare it over the month and the month before that to check for consistency, and then total your expenditure. Get down all your earnings and look at the difference. Are you making or losing money each month? How much can you save or how much debt can you clear? Try to get everything on here, including fuel for your car and how much do you need for food each week. Make sure you have enough to cover these basics. How much do you have left for your lifestyle, going out and having lunch, nights out, etc? Once you know all this, it will help you take control of it all and you can even set targets, goals, or dreams around it. You will know what's coming in, what's going out, and what you have to spare. You can even plan for the months ahead, including birthdays, dentist appointments, Christmas, and so on.

I truly believe money is the root of all evil. It causes greed, warfare, and even causes people to slaughter animals for parts of their bodies. All you need to do is worry about yours, forget everyone else's, and look after and control what you have. It will always come in, in some fashion. Even homeless people on the street have money coming to them. Just control where it goes and what on and keep enough so that you won't have any problems. If you truly need more than you can find, it may take time and hard work; but it's out there. Keep what you have saved and make sure you keep it growing. Use it to make more money rather than to spend on things that you don't need. Don't deprive yourself. If you truly want something you can get it, just make sure you know the reason you are buying it. You may need new clothing, new shoes. But how many pairs of shoes do you have and what condition are they in? Is it a need or a want? Will you be throwing out the old ones? Because if not, then you don't need them. It will be harder to lose money on needs over wants. Wants can break you, literally. Keep to the basics. You don't need everything, just the essentials.

Clutter can make you miserable. If you spend money on making your house nice and it increases the value of your house, then it could be worth it. If the money is going on your environment, plants, etc. and this helps make you happy, then go for it. Don't be oversold on stuff you don't need. Same as the other chapters. It's up to you what you do, and you can make the right decision. Just make sure you are aware of the consequences and the risks. Will it make you miserable or will it make you happy? Always a good question to ask yourself. If you really want something, then give it a month before getting it. If you still want it, then go for it. But ask the question first and make sure you have the right answer. Does it involve looking after you or taking care of yourself? That should be a high priority spend. Are you buying just to make you happier? Consider your emotional state when you are shopping? If you can wait a month and you don't want the item, then take that money and put it in your savings account. If you can't afford to save it, then you can't afford to spend it. If you save every time you would have spent, then you would end up saving a lot. If you can, then give back, give to charity, give to someone who needs it. For what is leftover or the extra, you can give and that will come back. If you invest and put money into companies, then you will earn interest on your money and the dividends back.

Don't always go with what you read, hear, or see. Make sure you follow the advice and guidance of a financial expert, such as a qualified, reputable financial advisor. The money will always come in, but can you control it going out? That is the key thing. There is enough money in the world for anyone to make a million. So, find yours, get yours, because you deserve it. It can be done as easy as investing a fixed amount of money each month rather than saving and then reinvest all interest earned and dividends and then letting it compound over time. You could set up a business, but make sure you know the return on investment, make sure you are doing something you love and will be passionate about. Because if you are not, then you will fail. Mark my words. You can't just have the passion. You will need to know what you are doing and have a plan to take the business to where you want it to go, and you will have to have the belief that it will succeed. So much that you have it as a vision. You can see it and you know exactly how it will go, how much it will make, when you will make it, where will it all come from, and then, where will you direct that flow. Will you reinvest it into your business? Will you take a percentage for marketing? Will you pay yourself a salary? Make it all clear as the clearer it is for you, and the more you see it and the more you go over it, then the more chance you have of making it happen. There is only a handful of ways you can build great wealth, creating a business, investing, high flying/successful career. I'm sure there are a few others, but these are the key ones, and most people that build wealth do so through investing. The sooner and earlier in life you can do it, then the more time you will have and the more wealth you can build. I think Warren Buffett started investing at seven years old or at least learnt about it; then it goes to show how he has become one of the wealthiest people on the planet as it seems as if he has been doing it the longest. The money will always flow; it will flow from the people who want it the least to the people who want it the most.

Chapter 6–Family, Friends, Relationships, and Parenting

This could be a hard topic, not just for you, but it is for me due to my personality type (see the last chapter for more on that). The parenting side I believe I have almost perfected as I have read quite a few books on the area, and it is my absolute passion and mission to be a great parent.

How well do you listen to someone when they talk to you? Do you make eye contact or are you looking at something else–a T.V. screen or a mobile phone? Are you just nodding your head, and do you glance at them now and again? Why would you do this when someone is taking the time to talk to you? How many friends do you have? How well do you listen to them? Everyone could improve on this topic. You could maintain eye contact. Some people might find it uncomfortable at first, but eventually, they will come to like talking to you even more because they know you're listening. They might even think you care, which is a great thing because then you can build a bond and they can then be there for you, which is a great thing to have. The more people you know and the more people that you have supporting you, then the more you will get out of life, from multiple angles with multiple benefits. If they have something important enough to say to you, then listen, show your true feeling and show compassion. This is a difficult skill to learn. It's a skill I learnt from talking to someone who was listening to me and this person even picked up on my lack of listening. I can honestly say it changed my life for the better. Also, people can see things better from the outside than you can from the inside. If you are being given an opinion on something or advice, never rule it out. Think about it, take it and say, "That's a good idea. I will think about it." Never rule it out, especially at first, as we automatically go on a defensive and a lot of times, we are wrong. So, be present, forget about everything else and stay focused on the current moment and keep eye contact. The information that someone shares with you could change your life. The first step is to listen, take it in, and then act on it. People in high authority roles always maintain eye contact when someone is talking to them. Just take a look at heads of state or royalty on television.

In terms of friends, do you think you will have more or fewer friends if you are there for people and listen to them and support them rather than just talking about you and your life? Can they rely on you? How about your partner? Can they talk to you? Make the most of every chance you get to listen to someone. You don't have to take their problems. You don't even have to worry about them. You can listen and completely forget about them if you want. It might be worth remembering the basics just in case you want to check up on them later or ask them about it, but it will never cause you any worry, unless they are in danger, in which case report it.

In terms of social media, I can't say I know much about it. But you can use it from the same point of view. Ask people how they are and check in on anything you have discussed. You can be there for them to talk to, but even better if you can arrange to meet in person and socialise in the real world. Share time with people. Have coffee or lunch with them and get out more. Get fresh air and enjoy life a little bit. Isn't it odd that sometimes spending time with family members is like spending time with people that you might not have anything in common with? Well, we are all humans—we breathe, eat, and sleep. Get to know your family. Spend time with them. Share good times and give them as much of your time as you can. Try to keep a balance though, don't spend so much time that you are off schedule with tasks. The more time with someone, the more you can be comfortable enough to unload to them, and this can then lead to arguments. You choose how much time, what works for you, what works for them, and if you are doing things together that you all enjoy. Everyone has a different idea of how long is right, so go with what you feel will give you a high score on the life cycle chart. You may not need to make any changes; you may not have any issues with how things are but just be aware of your score and how you can change it. If it helps you to improve, then great. If it raises your awareness and helps you to implement more time or more engaging times with your family, then great. Maybe eat together, go to events, do activities together; whatever you all enjoy. If you have kids, then great. If you can grow together and have fun together, then fantastic. Just remember, people don't always want to listen or even do what you want to do, so make sure you listen to them, their views and thoughts. Everyone has a different route to happiness. If kids are running around screaming having fun, is that a good thing or a bad thing. You can't handle the noise, then take yourself away from it. If they are having fun and enjoying themselves, then they are doing what you should be doing; you're missing out. You're trying to take that away from them, then you need to check yourself because you should be learning from them and listening to them; the same as everyone else. As they will end up not being happy because you're teaching them that being happy is wrong. You may be able to remember the feeling of being told off for running around screaming.

Once you have your dreams in place and achieve them, are you going to be jumping for joy, screaming with happiness, well there you go? Enjoy it and don't let anyone ruin it. Kids celebrate more and enjoy life more. Why don't we learn from them? Get your music on. Get in the right mindset. Get your emotions in check and have fun. This should be the biggest part of your life. Regardless, work, rest, and play should be fun, should be silly, and should be enjoyable. Let people judge you. I bet you will find more people liking you and wanting to have fun with you than you will find people judging you. So, let go. Let go of all this adult stuff of having rules and not drawing on the walls. It will wipe off and if it doesn't, then you should have used wipeable paint. Whose fault is that, the kids or yours? Everything comes back to you so don't blame anyone. Take responsibility and life will be a lot easier as you won't blame others and then you won't be so unhappy about it. Your kids are never really doing anything wrong; they are either doing something they have learnt from you or someone else and they don't really realise the consequences if there even is any. What you need to understand is that your kids, depending on their age, may not have fully developed brains yet and may not realise what is right, what is wrong, and so on. So, give them a break. Let them enjoy their childhood while it lasts, as you know what it is like once you become an adult.

What will happen if your kids become unhappy? How will that affect you and your family? You know the answer. I ask these questions throughout the book to stimulate your thinking. They are assuming you know the answer and you can use the question to draw it out and get the end result you want or use to support you in taking action and putting changes into place that will help to improve your way of life and your behaviour. When you improve your behaviour, then you will improve the results you get in life and the response and reactions that you get from others. Thoughts, feelings, behaviour, and reactions can all drive your life in one direction. So, bring it back to your thoughts, come to realise you are not always right about everything and your judgement of people may be wrong, and if it's negative, then is it driving a negative response from you and making your life less enjoyable and less fun. Get a positive mindset, find the positive in every situation, react to it and see how things go. Try it for a short time, a few days or a week, and see if your life changes in any way. How do you feel after doing it? How do you feel from always trying to be nice? How did people react to you? Do you think your life would be improved by this or do you think it will end up the other way? Do everything you can to get on with and support the people closest to you. They need you and one day you may need them. Don't make judgments on them or anyone else as this will be just opinion, and opinions are simply that–they are not true and not facts. If you have misjudged, then it will harm them, and it will harm you. Be nice, have fun, and enjoy life.

I know people and I know how they think, how they work, and why they do the things they do. What are we going to touch on? Well, let's delve straight in; jump in at the deep end! When you are in a relationship, what made you choose that person? Looks, personality, or something else? Their status? One thing that truly is important is what is their values and their mission. Now, I hope this doesn't cause you problems, but if their values and mission and dreams are different from yours, then you may be facing resistance; you may find things struggle to work. If you set them out individually and compare and they align, then you should be in a good place. This is something you want to find out early on about: what do they want, what are they about, and where do they want to go with their life? These can be some really basic dating questions that could help you identify the right person for you and for what you want; someone that can work with you and not against you. But what happens when you achieve those dreams or your mission? What happens if one of you changes their focus and direction? Then you could be in trouble. So, it's a good idea to review your values and mission and dreams with them and try to comprise on something that works for both of you, that will help you to grow together and to live together happily. Take it as time together–sit together, plan it, and communicate. Lay them out. If they don't align, can you support each other and still make it work? Make it clear where you both want to go, what you both want.

Say your partner wants to join the army and ends up being away a lot. Can you be supportive of that person and be there for them? They will love you so much more if you support them, and if you don't, then you could end up resenting each other. Now, if you don't want to support them, then maybe you are with them for the wrong reasons. Maybe you are just in it for yourself, in which case it may be time to consider things. You may not even have to think about it. You may naturally work well together and support each other. If you value being happy and the other person is depressed, then that could affect you and it could affect you a lot. Can you be there for them? Are they going to bring you down or can you bring them up? Will it really work if you are not on the same page? Can this person really find themselves or are they depending on you to make them happy? They should be bringing happiness in, not draining it out of you. Think about it, that could even be a barrier to you achieving your goals. Remember, if you aren't working together, then you will be working against each other–it's the yin and yang again. It's resistance and we know how that will turn out.

How do you set goals together? Well, you don't. You keep them
independent and then align them afterwards. Because if you
work on one person's goals, then it's not your life. It will be their
life and if things fall apart, you could be in trouble. Things could
go bad, really bad. So, set individual goals, missions and dreams
and then bring them together, work on them together, don't let
them divide you, work as a team to support each other, and
figure out a way that you can both succeed. Make your own
choices and be independent within the relationship. Go back to
the last chapters about planning out goals and the life cycle. Your
relationship may even be a part of these processes. So, that's
even more reason to keep them separate. You could even have
shared goals that you work on together afterwards or as part of
the whole plan. Think about happiness and what will make you
happy, and if the other person is happy, then you will be a strong
unit. Don't let your relationship take away your identity. You
should be able to find yourself quite quickly and quite easily.
Think back to your childhood and different stages of your life, as
a youngster, teenager, twenties up to your current age. What did
you enjoy? What brought you happiness? What are you proud
of? What regrets do you have that you can learn from? What can
you use to make sure you have values and how you can discuss
each other's past and share values based on that? What will
prevent you from success in any area of your life? Be it fitness,
diet, money, work, relationships, etc.? Remember, everyone's
plans, and values and life cycles will be different. This will help
you to identify you, find yourself, and be you, even in a
relationship. You might have a different cycle to everyone else.
You might have holidays in there. You might have your own
business. You might do charity work. Whatever is relevant to
you and whatever brings you a balance and supports your
relationship, do it.

Think about communication. You need to get your thoughts across, but it's all about you, which is what we want. But one big issue is we talk a lot and don't really listen enough. There's a range of different levels of listening. Think of the person that nods or says yes now and again and doesn't even make eye contact. Then have you had someone lock eyes with you when you are talking to them. They are taking everything in, a bit like when you are on a date, sat opposite them, having a meal. That should be the highest point. You feel uncomfortable, but you shouldn't. You should be learning that this is the way to listen, to be there for them, regardless of who it is and what they want. Work towards happiness for you and everyone you meet. I take that back. Don't work towards it, have it now and enjoy it. Take control. People talk and unload all the time. They talk about their problems and continuously ask, how did life come to that? Get rid of it, forget about it, and stop living in a different place, a different time zone. Pull yourself back to the present and don't even dare to start thinking about what might happen. It is important to be there for the other person, whether it's a partner, friend, or family member. Let them talk about their problems, help them to work towards getting rid of their problems. You don't have to take them and resolve them, just be there without this basic communication. What do you have? A relationship with very little feeling, with poor communication, maybe even broken language, with misunderstanding, or a lack of emotional support? Then you lack a stable relationship.

You're in a relationship, so relate like you're on a ship. Are you putting yourself before them? Look after yourself for sure, but give them something in return. Have you been there for them? If they don't support your dream or values (I'm not talking short term, I mean for life) then they don't care about you. Are they supporting you at work or are they moaning you work too hard?

Let them know you want their support. Then, is your life cycle balanced; is work high and family life low? Are you spending too much money or saving too much? Are they complaining about it? Are they grateful? Are they telling you how to live and running your life or do they share your values and work with you rather than against you? Do they want to be happy (because surely everyone does)? Make sure you review your lifecycle and values so things don't fall apart. You don't have to follow this, but use it as you wish to support you and what you want to do. You may want to pick bits out. You may want to use the whole thing or you may not bother with it at all because you may have everything in place. But I doubt it, as you wouldn't have even picked up this book. Use it to your advantage for your needs. As with anything, it is just opinions, so make your own choices. It's your life and you should live it, how you want to live, but live with happiness.

Aim to keep a balance, aim for longevity, try to live a slower, less stressed life, and aim for living the journey. Remember the tortoise and the hare. Have everything you want and take it, live your life.

So, how much detail will we cover on parenting, just really some basics to be honest with you? Each topic in the book, I have gone with that approach, as I want it to be a guide to support you in multiple areas of your life with pointers and tips to help you improve things. I won't be covering every age group and I will just look to go over some essentials based on what I have seen and what I have learnt. I may bring more in-depth titles on some of these topics in the future.

Number one, always be positive and enjoy every moment of parenting, no matter what. Kids drawing on the walls, pulling everything out of the cupboards, pushing buttons on the T.V., chucking food on the floor, anything that might bother you in the slightest, enjoy it. You have limited time with your kids, and it is disappearing second by second. If you get upset, bothered, angry with stupid little things, with your beautiful little baby, then you are doing two fundamental things wrong–you are breaking your bond with them and you are teaching them that it is okay to get angry, upset, and bothered over stupid little things. You are also teaching them that it's not okay to explore and have fun. Why? Because you don't want to pick up the food or the stuff they pulled out of the cupboard? How about suggesting they help and bond over that, make a game of it and have fun–double winner? You are having fun with both moments, making the mess and clearing it up. Can you laugh with them at the T.V. going on and off? Can you clean the wall off and can they help? Will they learn to tidy up after themselves? Think about these things. Can you and your baby enjoy simple things in life together and have a great time at home? Can you let go of the worry of things costing you money to repair? You earn more money every week. Can you earn more time with your baby and undo the damage of breaking a bond? I know which is easier for me.

Can you change your approach from what your parents taught you? Nothing will bring you more happiness in your life than your children, so give them back as much happiness as they give you. If you don't have kids, then having kids will be the best thing you ever do, I guarantee it! It will bring you great purpose and great value. So, give them that back. Use your support network, your family, the number one support network that you have. If they are not, then get them on your side. They should be there for you if you need them, and vice versa. Entertain your kids and make that the priority, every moment that you can, and be a part of it. Your life is their life and their lives are your life.

Take them out every week, even if it's free, especially if it's free, as that can be the best times–parks, beaches, walks, or take them to see family. How do you manage, live with, and enjoy times with your kids? Paramount is to keep them safe and healthy. Can you give your kids everything they want without any issues? Do they want two packs of crisps in a day? Why is that a problem? Are they having 10? Nope. Will two packs cause them any harm? Unlikely. Yes, cap a limit. Yes, they can eat dinner later. Are they happy or are they miserable and doing as you tell them because you think it's the right thing to do; because that's what everyone else does, or that's what your parents did? So, maybe do what they want and let them be happy if they are safe and it's not over the top. Moderation is the key to everything. Safety first, then happiness, enjoyment, and a great bond. What else do you need, food and water, of course?

This is for life in general, not just with your kids. Don't have any expectations of how you see the day going or your life. Because what happens if your expectations are not met? You envision your drive to work; it takes 10 minutes every day. You put everything in the car, head off out, down the road, around the corner and the road closed. Does it bother you? Yep, I reckon so. Why? Because you expected to be at work on time, now you will be late. Now you must think of another route when you were thinking about something else. Your thought pattern has been interrupted. Well, you know what, it doesn't matter. You are upset over nothing and you are making yourself miserable over nothing. Why? Because you have lost control. Your emotions have taken over control of your brain, and you are letting off steam. Well, rein it back, take control, and refuse to lose control. Keep your emotions in check, sit back in your car and chill. While you cruise around and enjoy your life, get to work late and everything will be better than usual, especially if your emotions are in check and you have taken back control. Think for the moment, live in the moment, and let the day come at you. Let the day flow by and enjoy it. Let your kids see you enjoying life, then they will too. Do you have to leave the park when you say so, or can they finish having fun for another five minutes? Will they get bored and then say they want to go? Let them take charge and there's a good chance they will grow up to be decisive, emotionally stable people. If you ask a question which is closed, such as are you ready to leave and they say no, then you must accept that. If you say when shall we leave, then they know it's happening, and they can help you decide. You can even negotiate. If you are leaving the house, you don't even have to say anything. You could just put on your jacket and shoes and see if they follow suit. People copy people, people very rarely listen to people, and people also like to listen to themselves. So, show, ask, but never tell. Keep your bond, keep your love and mutual respect, and life will be easier and happier. If you shout and tell them off, that's what they will learn. They learn from what they see from you.

Consider your tone and body language, just as much as your words. You can say whatever you want if it's in the right tone. This doesn't mean you should, though. Look at comedians. They rip into their audiences and get away with it, as they are using funny tones and body language. This, however, is not suitable for your kids. Your body language and tone can be very influential. They can see you more and pick up on the tone more and with ease of taking in the words. How you act and behave, they will pick up on it, and they will learn to be like you. So, be great, be nice, be happy, laugh, smile, and have fun. Give your kid's life, give them great times and enjoy them together. Have you ever bought something because someone told you to? Unlikely. Have you bought something because you have seen someone else with it? A lot of times. I guarantee it– shoes, cars, phones, watches; you name it. You would have seen it somewhere, on T.V., in an advertisement or in a film. People copy people. Show your kids greatness and they will be great. Show them fun and they will have fun and show them happiness and they will be happy.

Don't lose control. You don't have to give them everything they want in life; you can still have an aspect of discipline. Just remember, you don't have to punish your kids. Are they actually naughty or are you just upset? Can you talk to them and show them the right way? Can you reward and praise for the good things which will encourage good behaviour? Can you demonstrate and lead an example of good behaviour? Don't discipline and over punish, encourage, and praise. Forget making them sit on a step. This will break and ruin your bond with your child. It will break down your relationship. Half the time, they may not have even been naughty, they just haven't done what you wanted them to do. Sure, you can't have your kids going around hitting other kids. So then take a bit of responsibility and talk to them, and you know what, for all the times, you joined them in pulling stuff out of cupboards, making a mess, having fun and working together to tidy up, you will have a great bond. So, when you talk to them about hitting, then guess what? They will probably listen. The good thing is that you are interacting with them and having a great time with them, thereby creating good memories.

I assure you, I'm not the perfect parent. I'm not even sure if there is such a thing. Remember, no one or nothing is perfect. But if that was the case, I will aim and strive to be it and I will always aim for the fundamental basics of being happy, my kids being happy, safe and enjoying their lives. I will aim to give them everything I can, accommodate their needs, and make sure they are always entertained. You can do this too. You just have to reset your mindset, be aware of it, and make basic little changes, such as letting go of the worry and enjoying life no matter what. Because life will go by with or without you, and you have very little control over anything in the world, including parts of you. For example, when you need to go to the toilet or when you sleep, sometimes your body will take over and you will have to go to bed because you're tired. But you can control your mind. They say we use 10% of it. I believe that is the conscious part. Well, take control of a little bit more, including your emotions. Be there for your kids, put your hand on their back if they are upset, unless they kick out, then give them a little space to think about things and be upset. They are learning about their emotions, but be just close enough that they know you are there for them. Within seconds, they can change and go back to having fun. But be careful and tread lightly as they may get upset again. So, back off a bit again if needs be; it's a basic law of attraction. Putting them on a step is too much space because they are on their own out of the room. The space should be within the same room and it should be their own choice. By all means, suggest they have a minute. Why can't it be on the sofa, cuddled up to you and sharing it together? Do you need space? Are you upset? You can do the same. You can take five minutes out. It can be at any time. Don't leave your kids alone, but if you experience something and can't take control of your emotions, then give yourself a break. It could be in the car, before you go in the house, maybe in a lay-by, or you could go to the toilet and just sit there for a minute.

Safety, happiness, enjoyment and fun. What more could you want? Add more if you wish but keep it basic? Enjoy spinning around the front room, dancing, splashing in puddles, going down slides and jumping in ball pits. Now, not on your own or maybe if you can get away with it, but ideally with your kids. Have lots of fun with them and they will have fun too. What could be better? Take yourself back to your childhood. What were the best moments? What memories do you have? Was it going to places, spending time with family and friends, going to a movie? Think about the memories you want to build for your kids. Do you have any bad memories that you have from growing up and how can you avoid putting your kids through the same? You may not be able to afford to buy them something that they want, but do you really need to tell them that? Did you grow up with your parents saying you can't have something because they can't afford it? How can you work around this? Can you tell them that they can have it next time or help them to save pocket money to obtain the thing that they want? How can you use it as an opportunity for your child to learn? Maybe they can learn that they don't have to have everything that they want. Can you show them this by not having everything yourself? What do you get from having very little? You may have a need; you may have a want? Very rarely will that need or want to relate to happiness.

Chapter 7– Happiness, Tired, Bored and Hungry

I believe this can stem back to your upbringing and that most people spend the bulk of their time either being happy or unhappy. Their mood may change, but they always come back to their normal state. I believe I am lucky enough to be on the happy side most of the time due to having a great upbringing and I have always appreciated the simple things in life. I felt like generally I was spoilt as a child, even though we didn't have a lot, and I feel this has helped me to realise you don't need all the material things in the world to make you happy. I have come to realise simple things like tiredness can affect your happiness and I'm sure they call sleep deprivation the worst form of torture. Let's not torture ourselves, let's do the opposite.

Happiness - How happy are you? Do you have any problems? Well, that can depend on your emotional state. If you are happy, then it's easier to laugh at life's problems. If you are in a bad place, then they will only pile on top and add to your issue. But are they the problem or is it something else? Of course, it's something else. You just haven't dealt with it and the emotion has built up and then you are letting it out all over the place, on any little thing which really isn't an issue. Then you can't take responsibility and take control of everything and make your life perfect. It's just not a short-term job. It's like a plant that needs constant looking after. And constant planning to make sure your emotions are in check and then you can sail through the day with ease.

Go back over each chapter, get the key points in place including, values, goals, dreams, etc. This will help you develop a plan to have more purpose, more drive, something to live for, something to work for, and a real sense of direction. Listen to people. Be more about them and they will be more about you. Be in the moment, live the moment, forget having things and wanting things, take life, and have life. Drive forward for the moment. Forget people's views on what you should be and line out what you want and what your expectations are. If you live for someone else's views or dreams, then you will lose a lot. You will waste it all. Make it yours and don't regret it. If you strive to do something and have something, will you enjoy it or is it short term? Setting something to work towards can bring the enjoyment of the journey, but if you get to it and achieve it, then review it as you may then no longer have a purpose or dream to live for, and you need that. Consider current happiness, not as a result.

You can be happy in any situation. Be happy with it and accept it as life. Get in the right frame of mind, and if something knocks it back, it will only be temporary. Your state of happiness will always return, providing just that for you. If you are not happy all the time, then that is what you will return to. We are always going to be whatever we think we are and nothing else unless we change our mindset. Gratitude, this one single thing, will bring you so much happiness and not directly from being grateful, but as a knock-on effect. If you start a day with being grateful for something, anything–the weather, the daylight, the car you have to get you to work in the rain, anything–then keep it going throughout. It will help your mindset to focus on the positives. It will help you look at what you do have and it will help you to be a state of mind that will maintain a happy day, and a happy day every day means a happy week, and every week means a happy month, and a year works you towards a happy life. Money or things–for example, cars and houses–won't bring you happiness, only temporarily. Think about getting the latest phone. Has that ever made you happy? Then the next time you change it, did that make you happy? So, when you change it, did the old one-stop making you happy. Sure it did, because you were no longer grateful for it, so you sold it or chucked it away or threw it in a drawer. If it was broken and you were grateful for it, then you would have taken it to be repaired, unless it was cheaper to replace, of course. Get the balance right, remember. Be grateful for everything–fresh air, the meal you're having that night. Are you in good health? You stop being grateful, then you could easily lose these things, or they could be discarded by you (neglected). Are you eating junk food suddenly because you don't appreciate your health?

Take care of your environment as we covered earlier–keep it tidy, clean it. Look after yourself, get some form of exercise. Review your life balance. Why would you make yourself sad by looking at the things you want and the things you maybe can't even have? That's why it makes you happy to buy it because you can't have it and it makes you sad, so buying it solves that problem, whether you can afford it or not. If you are single and unhappy about it, how are you going to find a partner? They don't want to be with someone that is unhappy. So, get your mind in the right place and focus on the present. That person might be talking to you and you might not be listening to them. They might have sat on the train opposite you, but you are too busy reading this book and not taking a day off to just chat with people. Find out where they are from and what they do for a living and listen to them. Because if you give them half a chance, they will open up to you and start talking, and you don't even have to say much. Just keep eye contact, prompt them for more information now and again, ask questions, and you are there; you are in the present moment. The phone is off, television is off, the book is down.

What about your kids? Are they screaming at you? Why? Where did they learn it? Did you scream at them at some point for being too noisy? Then stop it. Don't shout at them, shout with them. Scream with them and see how much fun it is. Why are you telling them to stop? It's fun. Why can't you do it and have fun too? Because your parents told you to not do it or people might look at you? So what, you're having fun and you're happy and so are your kids. They will learn what they see from you, not what they hear. You shout at them and tell them off. They will learn to shout at you. Show them and they will follow.

How many people go to work and enjoy it? Well, I'm lucky enough to be in that position and I would recommend doing everything in your power to get in that position, no matter how long it takes, as it will be worth it and you won't feel like you're working ever again. Go back to that chapter if you need to.

I can honestly say it took me 36 years to find permanent happiness. I spent a lot of my time being happy for just short bursts–maybe an hour here or there, a day, a week, maybe even a month if I was lucky, but never all the time. I felt like something was wrong with me because I wasn't happy all the time. I felt like I was missing out and everyone else was happy all the time. Wow! How self-absorbed was I? I can see now that most people are not happy like I thought they were, because they show it when you see them and talk to them. If you listen to them, then you will find out the truth that they all have problems. Everyone has something wrong in their lives and most of them just want someone to talk to about it and they are all in search of being happy when it's right in front of them. Be grateful for everything you have, establish your values and dreams to give yourself purpose, and then enjoy the ride. Find the right mindset for the day, prepare for the day, be ready to take on the world, and have your eyes open to see the opportunity out there. Plan it out. How much time do you need and what do you need to do? Get it down on paper, which things must be done, and which ones don't matter. Got your motivations? Great, run with them.

Can't find your goals, dreams, and values, then spend time researching them online. What do other people value or dream off, ask them, get as many ideas as you possibly can. How did I find it? I followed this. I knew what I wanted, and I stopped wasting time. I stopped wasting my life watching television and online. I did the things that I wanted to do that worked towards my dreams and I kept going. I did it when I wasn't enjoying it and worked out why. Sometimes you need a rest. Balance your time, do everything for your dreams within the balance, and work towards them daily, if not weekly. They will come a lot quicker than if you sit around watching television or wasting time on things you don't really care about and just do for the sake of it or out of routine. Go cold turkey if you can and cut out these habits as though they were drugs taking away your life. Then look at all the great things in your life which are maybe not even great, but they should be. You just haven't realised it. Be grateful, every day and for everything, I can't stress the importance of that enough, as it will truly help you get there. If you are grateful for your family, they will make you so happy when you next see them. Remember, it's a journey and not a destination. You don't want to get there and then go home. You want to enjoy it all the way until the end.

Take control and tell yourself you will be happy. You can get up for work and have expectations of the day, but then you have set yourself up to fail because your kettle might break, you may have forgotten to wash your clothing, you might encounter roadworks causing delays, and so on. What, are you going to let these things ruin your day or are you going to be happy and then just ride those waves? Let them come at you one after the other and then wait for the big one where you can ride it all the way into the shore. You can take each one as it comes and accept it. So, there's traffic. You will be late for work. That could actually be a good thing. Will your boss be shouting at you because they are in the wrong state of mind for the day? Do they have underlying issues with something in their life, so they have decided to vent it towards you? Let it bounce off. They can go on and on, but you can keep your happiness because you have full control over it. Be grateful for that person, as you are getting paid money just to be there and to listen to them. You know that you haven't done anything wrong. Well, maybe you didn't plan your journey good enough, but it's in the past and you're in the present. Sure-fire one out of the five working days you may get issues, but the world is out there and moving at a pace. Get out there and ride through it. Look after yourself, get the right amount of sleep for you; not what I say or anyone else. What you feel is right. Educate yourself but only if you want to and learn everything that you want to, to take you forward. Give back, help others, but only if you can and only if you want to. It may make you feel great for its one step towards greatness.

But you may already be there. How you feel is how you will be; so, feel great. Look after yourself first, then everybody else. If you are on a plane with your kids, they tell you to put your mask on first. Because if you stop breathing, then you can't help them. So, you first, then everyone else. Be healthy, keep healthy. Then, when people ask you how you are so happy or why, you don't have to give them this book. You can tell them or show them. They might want to listen if they are asking you. But it could be better to show them. They will notice you are happy way before you tell them you are. They may not want to know. They may already be happy with their lives and you will be fine with that because you can listen to them and you may even value them. Also, you have your direction and it doesn't have to cross paths with anyone else unless you want it to. You will do it how you want, and if they understand, then they will be happy for you. But remember, they may struggle to find happiness. But if they do, then you will see it and it will bring you even more happiness. Just knowing that doesn't affect you. Take the first ten minutes of your day, sit up in bed and have that place or sitting in your car or wherever you want as a place for you to prepare; it might be in the shower or even on the toilet. Just take ten minutes and think about how you would like your day to go. Note what you want to get out of it; well, maybe not in the shower. You could use a note app on your phone, but, of course, wait until you get out the shower first. Take some time and the bulk of the ten minutes to think about what you are grateful for and make a list of just three 3 things. You can repeat these at any point, but today, what are the three for today? There is no wrong or right. It can be anything and I assure you it will make your day a little bit better. As you will have a true appreciation for things and then eventually, you will have a true appreciation for life.

You won't feel the constant need to change things or upgrade things, as you will have everything you need. Don't let people throw you off with this. They may be making comments or judging you on things, well that doesn't matter. I know it can hurt if you feel like someone you love is judging you, but just put it down to lack of understanding. They may not understand, or they may not have learnt the same things in life as you, so they simply just don't really know. You can't blame people for not really knowing. Don't feel like you must explain to them or tell them either. Just acknowledge what they are telling you might help and remember to listen. But if you feel and know that you are doing the right thing, then let it bounce off you and continue to be happy. Create a happiness force-field and let all that kind of stuff just bounce off you. Being happy should be number one on your list and doing everything in your life that contributes to it. Have this mindset every morning. What will make your day perfect or as near as possible? Remember, there is no perfect, so if that's what you really aim for, then it won't be achieved. Just aim to be happy and to enjoy your day, that can't be so hard, I know the world will throw a lot at you and try to stop this from happening, but all you have to do is approach the world with the right mindset by getting in the right emotional state before you start the day. Be grateful–I can't stress this enough–see how you want it to go, feel how you are in yourself, and prepare with some music if it helps. Maybe even put some headphones in and block out the world for ten minutes. Have music that will make you feel great, music that you love, music that will bring you up and make you feel ready for the day. Tackle and take the world head-on and with happiness, because there is only one of you out there and the world needs you, people need you, and they need you to be happy. Just like sadness, happiness spreads and it spreads like a viral video online. If you are happy, then everyone around you will be happy. Bring happiness into every room that you enter and take it with you when you leave.

I chose the title of this chapter because it's a common complaint that I have heard, and I can even recall saying when I was younger. I don't want to target age groups, but I feel it might be more of a younger age group that believes this based on the judgement of solely myself and the people I have heard it from. Now, it may not be all three of them at once (fatigue, boredom, and hunger), you might just be affected by one of them. But I'm sure I have been affected by all three in the past and I would be amazed if someone hasn't. Even having kids, you can see a lot of the time if they are acting up, then it can come back to these three things–not all the time but a lot of the time. So, if they have eaten recently, and you can see they are not really tired by looking at them, then are they just bored? Do they just want something to do? I bet it is, and if you ask them if they want to do something, then they will think about and most lightly take you up on it. You can even ask them what they want to do. So, the next time they are doing something you don't approve of, such as smashing things, drawing on things, then test it out. Then, if they were acting up, crying or whining, and you find them something to do, guess what? They will be happy. It's that simple. I will cover this more on the chapter about parenting and the results that lead on from the happiness chapter.

Think about yourself. Are you bored, tired, or hungry? Or is it something else? It normally leads back to those things. If you have had a long day at work, you might be tired physically. If you don't feel great when you wake up, then you may not have slept well. Did you have a power nap during the day? Are you mentally tired from looking at a screen all day? Can you get a power nap in? Can you solve these problems and make your day better? Because if you stay on top of them, then you won't have many other problems. You should be pretty much okay. You might have niggles, a bad back or some other health complaint, but do what you can to solve them. Can yoga help? Do you need medicine, or do you just need a nice warm shower or bath and some sleep? Get a solution. Don't moan; fix it. The less you moan, the quicker you can fix it because the body will believe whatever the mind thinks.

We have covered food in a previous chapter, but let's revisit some of the ideas previously discussed. So, do you remember the key points? The right number of calories, the right nutrients and minerals. Do you have the calories you need? You wouldn't put diesel in a Ferrari, so why do you put junk in your body? Value yourself and your body and do everything you can to take good care of it and look after it. Prepare everything you need for your day. Have your pots, carrots, tomatoes, cucumber, cheese, etc. and even chocolate as a one-off now and again. Be good and go for as pure as possible dark chocolate and limit the number of squares that fit into your calorie count. If you can satisfy your hunger, then we have one less issue and one step forward towards greatness. It can help you to work to your optimum level and it can help your emotional state.

People do eat with their emotions and they do eat to make themselves happy. People even go as far as eating and drinking foods that they don't need, and I have done it myself, saying I need a coffee when really all I need is water. If you have the food readily available, then you may be less likely to buy junk food and this can help to satisfy that hunger. You could go the whole day without food. You may not feel great if you do and may even feel tired. I wouldn't recommend it, but your body is able to do it, especially if you ate well the day before and have had plenty of water. The point is, you don't need to moan about being hungry. If you're not eating or you're not eating right, then you won't have the energy you need. So, get the fuel to get the fats and the carbohydrates and a bit of protein, but not as much as you may think.

You can also experience boredom. Picture it, you get home from work; you hang your jacket up; you take your shoes off, and you shut down from work. It's all put-away and down with for the day. You make dinner and clear up. What now, it's seven at night, maybe earlier, maybe later. Do you go to the gym, do you watch T.V.? Do you sit and scroll through social media or play games? What are you doing? Are you valuing your time? Are you doing these things because you're bored? Do you watch television every night? Do you get home and watch it from 7 to 9 o'clock? Maybe two hours a night, every day, 5 working days. This would be 10 hours a week or 40 hours a month? That's equivalent to a whole working week. What could you do with a whole working week? Maybe television is boring and you are just stuck in a routine? Could you do something productive? Could you set up a business in your spare time, learn a language, an instrument, could you write a book? Well, I did and you're reading it. You could even work a part-time job and earn some extra money. Overall, you can gain a lot of time. You don't have to do it every night, just maybe when you are bored and want to feel some fulfilment and have some purpose to your life. You could even do charity work one night a week. You may have kids and may have to put them to bed and not really have the time to get bored. But I'm sure you get it. At some point, then, if you do, have just one thing you can turn to that will give you a bit more purpose and something you can work towards. You may not need to. You may not want to, but it's an idea if you feel you might need it. You could even go to college one night a week and do a part-time course. Meet friends for dinner or invite them or family around. It's a good opportunity to work on the cycle and build up an area you may be low on.

So, we have covered boredom, hunger, and fatigue. Remember to try and get those naps in. That can be hard, but try to work them into your day and see if it helps. You may not want to take anything from this, but if you can benefit from one point, then great. If you can benefit from multiple points, then even better. So, work on these points if it helps. They could help you get into a good emotional mindset and be less grouchy for the day and more focused, more driven towards something and a little bit more positive with how we feel in general. Food can also affect this if you are having high sugars, which could bring you up and then crash back down later in the day. So, be aware of that. Plan it out and prepare to prevent it. Go with what works for you and the foods you like and limit the junk food to when you really need it.

Do you need to bring yourself up a bit and make yourself a little bit happier, and are you willing to risk it with junk food that could be doing more long-term damage? Look after that Ferrari and keep it gleaming bright red. Get good fuel in it and clean and looked after. People will look on at you and you will turn heads. It may be raining outside but you can still have a good colour to your skin just from eating right; just from having the right vitamins and getting enough of them. You don't need a sun shower or spray tan; you need to eat right. Two carrots a day carry enough carotene to improve your complexion. Don't overdo it as too much can cause other side effects. Eat them raw if it helps or try sweet potato, tomatoes, or even spinach. Whatever works for you. I'm not giving you anything new here, just some fundamentals that not many people follow these days. Get some rest, eat right, and fulfil your time.

Bad habits can take over and become consuming. We're wired that way. A high percentage of what we do is a habit, and we do it because it saves us from having to think too much. The mind is taking in millions of information every second, so it lessens the burden on the brain to do things on autopilot, as it were. So, we don't think so much about what we are eating or what we are doing. You ever drive for a period of time and not really notice part of the journey as your mind drifted off? That's like autopilot. Make the same breakfast every day without even thinking about what you want? Pick the same stuff off the shelf in the supermarket? Again, all on autopilot. Shops love it. You keep going back to the same place and buying the same things without even thinking.

What can help break these habits? Well, first being aware of them. You can't change anything without being aware of it first. Then what, look after your mind, rest, sleep, meditate, break from screens, a break from people, a break from work, a break from music, and so on, then use it. Use your mind but for things that will help it develop, learn and grow. Read, take new courses, try new things, even try basic games like sudoku and chess. Do something hands-on with practical thinking, such as drawing or building Lego. Then start looking at your life as a big picture but reflect on all the little things; for example, do you want to drink coffee every day, do you want to eat the foods you are eating or go to the places that you are going to or even spend time with the people you are spending time with? Take a bit of reflective time. This can be done during your ten minutes in the morning, but it's not really needed every day. If that might work for you, you could think about the little things in your day–like what do you want to do, eat, drink; who do you want to see, how are you going to feel, and so on? People write a list to shop at the supermarket, so why can't you write a list of what you want from your day and what you will do and where your time, money, energy and everything else will be going. Just by looking after yourself that little bit more and looking after your mind, you should see some great benefits and hopefully start to see life from a slightly different perspective. Things will hopefully get easier, more fun, and more enjoyable. Learn to laugh everything off and learn to enjoy every moment and every day. Take notice of your emotional state and if it isn't the place you want to be in, then take five minutes out of your day, take a breather. A smoker would take five minutes to go outside and smoke. All they are doing is taking time out from the day and everything that is going on. So, do the same; take five-minutes breaks, even if it is going to the toilet or sitting in your car. Take that time when you need it and get a bit of a recovery to get your emotional state of mind into the place you want it to be before going back out there to the world and taking it all on and enjoying your time with everyone.

Chapter 8–Cause and Effect, and NLP

I learnt about this topic after realising that I was the main cause
of any of my problems in life and everyone else is the cause of
their own problems. The sooner you can get on board with that,
no matter how hard it is, then the sooner you can take control.
For if you take ownership of a problem rather than blaming
others, then you can resolve it. If you leave the blame on others,
then you can't do anything about it and you are giving them full
control over your problem. Take control and own your problems,
destroy them, and move forward.

The cause-and-effect principle say, for every cause, there is an
effect and for every effect, there is a cause. What does this
mean? Everything you think about, the way you behave and
everything you do, creates an effect. So, what causes you to
behave, think, and act in the way that you do? Because they
cause the effect if you change the causes and you will have a
different effect. So, if you are unhappy, depressed, sad, angry,
then you can change that by looking at the cause. Change your
actions and you will change your life. Change your thoughts and
you will change your actions. Life has no such thing as luck. You
make your own life and your own future. We choose everything
that we have in life, where we live, where we work, what we do,
and the people we spend time with. You have control of it all and
you can change it all in an instance. Take control of cause and
effect and you can take control of your mindset, your happiness,
and your life. Everything in your life is a result of your actions.
The decisions you make (the cause) will result in the result of
what you have (the action). This can cover everything including,
your wealth, your friends, your relationships, your mindset,

happiness, sadness, and so on. You can change your life just by changing how you think and then acting on your new thoughts. You can be happy just by thinking about it; it's that simple and that easy. How long it will last is up to you. It could last forever if you want it to.

So, what about other areas, work, finance, etc? Well, you can be successful in these areas and any others, including parenting, relationships and so on, just by being aware of what we are doing and making the right decisions, leading to making the right actions and the great end result. How do we make the right decisions? Well, you can look at other people and emulate them. Do you know someone that is always happy, someone that has a great relationship, lots of friends and lots of money? What did they do, how did they get to that point, and can you do it too? It may not be as easy as that sounds, you can't just do what they do. You will have to look at each area, such as how often they do it, their values, their drive, habits, time dedicated to the cause. If you do what you always did, you will get what you always got, right? So, if you do what someone else has done, then you could get what they have got. Did you get your job by chance or did you apply for it and have an interview? Did you get your house by chance or did you speak to someone, then rent or buy it? Nope, you thought about it and acted on it. Nothing happens by chance. You have to go out and get it. Everything happens for a reason. If it's good, then take it. If it's bad, then ride that wave and if you fall off, then get back on the board. Keep riding it as things will change and more opportunities will come.

Take risks, take lots of risks, and see how many you regret. I don't ever remember regretting taking a risk. The fear is worse than actually taking the risk and then the end result is usually great. The way you act and react will affect how you feel, how you behave, and vice versa, the way you feel and behave, will affect the way you act. This has a knock-on effect and can shape your life. Your thoughts produce the cause, your life is reflected in your thoughts. If you think happy, then you will be happy. If you spend your day around negative people, then you could end up being negative. If you watch the news and it's all bad news, then that can affect you. Your thoughts are you and they affect your whole life and how you see things. Everyone lives differently and sees everything differently. So, try to stay open-minded, try not to be influenced by others, the news and what you see; try to lead. Be positive and take charge of your life. You have full control over how you feel, think, and act; in which case, you can live your life exactly how you want to live it.

The first step is to be aware of it, which we have just done. We have found awareness and learnt about it. Then think and think a lot. Your first thoughts are normally wrong. You see something and then you instantly think, but do you challenge that thought or just go with it. Do you even need to think about it? Will it just bring you down? Can you move on and use that time for something else? Can you look at the good side of it and just enjoy life? Until you are aware of it, you are probably making decisions and choices based on how you have learnt, seen, and developed over time; barely thinking about it and operating on autopilot. You can unlearn these things or, better still, learn new ways of being and acting. You may have learnt from parents, friends, teachers, and work colleagues. They all had a bearing on you as a person and how you are. We only know what we see and learn. You may have even learnt from watching television or reading. So, how do we make these changes? Ask yourself. How do my thoughts affect my life? How do I see things and people? How can I change my thoughts on these things? Do they matter? How can I see it in a positive way? Who can I be like? Who can I act like? Who is the example of what I want to be like? Can I spend time with them and learn from them? Nothing is random; see it for what it is. Shape your life around it and enjoy it. Whatever your ambition is, it can be achieved. The first thing you need to do is to believe that it can be achieved. See it and envision it. Then live it and do everything you can to get it. Dream about it, plan it, learn about it, and bore people by talking about it and not stop going on about it. Be so passionate about it that it drives people mad. Dedicate your life to it if it's something you want that bad and will get you to the point of living your dream. Find out the barriers and work out how to get past them. Find out what others have done to get to that point that you want to get to and then spend as much free time on it as you possibly can. This, too, can drive it forward. Take action and just, quite simply, go for it. What have you got to lose? What could be better than chasing your dream? If you spend ten years trying to get there and you fail, will you give up or will you try a different approach? Be relentless and don't give up.

Review what you want as the years go by and your life develops as it may naturally change, which isn't giving up. It's changing your goals based on your life, needs, and wants. Whatever you do, keep going and keep on track to your purpose. Just don't let it pull you away from enjoying it. If you're not having fun anymore, then it may be worth having that review time, that reflective time, to decide if it's still what you want. Revaluate your life, your dreams, your values, your goals, and your mission. Take some downtime and think about everything and decide on what you want, need, and what will be best for you and your life.

The Neuro-Linguistic Programming (NLP) model is a representation of information communicated to us and information we communicate, including the way we act in our behaviour and how we see things, perceive them, understand them, or even believe them to be. Whatever we see, hear, or even feel, we do so in a way that is affected by our beliefs, values, and memories. We don't take in all the information that is communicated to us as our brains can't cope with all the information. We also don't always see, hear, or feel it in the way it may have been intended to be communicated to us, and we can also end up with a distorted view of it through how we perceive it. This information will then affect your internal state and wellbeing, your mindset and even your happiness. For example, if you see that someone has left a mess in the house, it could upset you as it looks untidy or you may have to clear it up. That could be your belief on how to deal with it, so your happiness is being affected by the external factor. It could then affect how you felt about the person that left the mess and you may then have a link of unhappiness towards them when you see them. This could even affect how you behave towards them or even how you are when greeted with this sort of situation. So, how do you prevent this unhappiness; not just with this situation, but with any situation?

Firstly, consider your initial thought. Your human instinct is to see it how it is and to go with your first thought. So, if something that causes you any kind of unhappiness, rather than accepting it and being unhappy, challenge yourself on it and question how you see it, or what you have heard or how you feel about it. It is okay for you to be wrong about something. In fact, it is great if you are wrong about it. If you notice you are wrong, challenge it and get rid of that unhappiness before it takes over. Does the person who left that mess have the same values as you? Probably not. Did they have the same education, upbringing, etc.? Do they have the same beliefs? Unlikely. Are you ever messy? Have you done this? Most likely. Would it be easier to tidy the mess and be happy than being unhappy? Have you seen the whole picture? Did they have to leave in a hurry because a family member was in the hospital? Have you got all the information? Would it be better to focus on you and what makes you happy rather than what makes you unhappy? If this is going to affect your behaviour, then what is the knock-on effect? Are you not going to get on with this person now and lose a friend? Are you going to let them have a lower opinion of you because of it?

We are presented with so much information that there is no way we can take in all the right things to be able to see everything how it is. We can only really take up to five bits of information at one time, so the rest gets ignored and isn't taken into account. Try to take yourself away from the issue or problem, think about how you feel, are you sad, angry, depressed, etc.? Turn away from the issue, go to a different room, different place, imagine you are somewhere else or someone else and you are doing something different, or even in the room with yourself and seeing you act or respond to it. How would you act if there was a stranger next to you or your grandmother? Would you act the same way? Would you still let it upset you? The key thing I'm trying to get across here is not all the science behind it or the theory. The point is everything we see, hear, and feel every day will affect us. It can make us happy, sad, or depressed. It may even push you to dark places or even places of complete euphoria. Do you want to give up control of your body, behaviour, mindset, emotions to everything you see, hear, and feel? Or do you want to take a bit of control over yourself? So, being aware of it in the first place, it will help you and then trying to change the habits that you have built over time will be the next part. Keep that awareness and consider how you will deal with things. You could have something that you turn to when you are presented with a situation that upsets you. You could use it as a cue to make yourself a drink, coffee, etc. and only do that during the day when you are presented with a situation. I wouldn't recommend cake or high-calorie foods as this could present the start of an eating disorder. Whatever upsets you, get yourself away from it. Keep the understanding that you could be wrong.

Someone cutting you off at a junction whilst driving might be rushing to the hospital with their pregnant wife. Someone getting angry with you over something trivial could be, and most probably is, doing so because they have some other issue going on in the background. Put yourself first, put your happiness over everything, as there is nothing more important than you, your family, and friends being really happy. This should be top of the list of what you want in life and nothing and no one should be able to affect that. Life is happening for you, not to you. You are here to enjoy it and make the most of it. Utilise every moment. If bad things happen, it's normally an opportunity for you to cease upon to learn from, develop from, and to become a better person, an opportunity to become stronger and carry less fear because you have learnt to deal with the situation. You would have experienced the pain from it and survived it. Why wouldn't you want to be happy? Why can't you get upset with something? Well, you can. Sure, if you want. But I very much doubt many people want that, and if you are happy and enjoy life, then you will live a more fulfilled life. You will reap the benefits of everything that comes with it, including success through great relationships, work, personal growth, and development, and even finance. But most importantly, you will have very little regrets and great memories, great experiences and great people in your life. This should be the goal, the dream, and your ambition. But again, who am I to tell you? Erase that part and fill it with your

own words of what you want and what you believe is right for
you.

Chapter 9–Achieving Greatness, Taking Action, Making Big Moves and Doing What You Want.

Greatness is whatever you want it to be in your eyes; how you see it. I have found mine once in being a dad. I am still looking for other ways to be great, including trying to help as many people as I can in life. I implemented taking action on other areas that I wanted to excel in by getting home from work every night and working until late at night on whatever project it is that I wanted to focus on for my mission. In making big moves, if you want to do something great, then you may have to take a risk. It is up to you to gauge how much risk you will take and balance it against the reward.

So, you have a goal and you want to achieve something, such as setting up a business, losing weight, learning a language, or even writing a book, but you can't seem to get moving. You're stuck on the couch, scrolling through your phone or binge-watching. You know what I mean, the constant watching of Netflix, show after show. The timing is counting down and the next episode is starting. Hell, you may not have even noticed. They all seem to blur into one or you had your face in your phone while the show is running in the background. Maybe it's YouTube; one video has finished, and you have made it onto something completely different, and you are lost down the wormhole. Or, the newest one which seems to be the endless stories on snap-chat. Well, I praise you if you are reading this, for you have made it this far in the book and took yourself away from the screens to learn something. You have your goal. You know what it is. If not, then what do you like, what do you want, what embodies your dreams and values, and then, how can you get it and what do you need to do? These are just a few questions you should be asking yourself. Then you want to plan out how long it will take, how much time do you need, and how much of a priority it is?

If you only have one goal, then you have a lot more chances in achieving it. Clear away all the others and then nothing will distract you from it. Even if you list 20 goals and then just pick out the top three and focus on the main one for the next year or so. So, let's say it's a language. You would need to learn at least 500-600 words; on average, two words a day for the next year might get you there, but it's never that simple. You will need to fully immerse yourself in this goal. You work your day; you spend time with family, and you do all the housework. If you need a power nap, take it and time it; no more than 20 minutes. If you need a rest, a bit like a short lunch break or tea break like you would at work, then do that. But it has to be planned into your day, then you have whatever time is left, be it 30 mins, one hour or whatever, you will need to find that. I know that it can be a big task for anyone if you have kids or are even a single parent. Trust me; I really know. I'm there and I'm scrapping for every second to fit everything in. That time every day is there for you–for your priority, for your goal, for your dream, to live your values and give you a little bit more purpose. Now, don't get me wrong, you may not have a purpose; everyone needs a purpose. Because if you don't, then you leave yourself at risk of wanting to end everything. If you have kids, then you have a great purpose, even parents, friends and so on, a job that helps people. You can even find other areas to gain purpose, such as helping people, looking for nothing in return; maybe even charity work, volunteering, and so on. But you need one little thing more than any of that and that is a purpose for you–a goal for you, a dream for you. What are you waiting for? Find it, get it down on paper, and plan it. Then commit that time as a priority and do it. It will be up to you how much time–it might be 10 minutes a day, one hour a week. Whatever it is, you have to do it completely for you. It has to be completely your choice and it will be something you will enjoy doing and will have a great result that will make you happy. This is your one chance to be completely selfish, and if anyone goes against you, then you will explain to them what it means to you, how it will make you happy. All you want from them is to support you, and if they don't want to support you, then you will do it anyway, as it will make you happy and then you can share that happiness with them. You don't need to share it with anyone, as most people will worry or look for fault in a way of trying to protect you. Well, you don't want protection as you have a plan and you are doing what you want for once in your life–not what your boss wants, not what your parents want, and not what your kids or partner wants. Tell them to get on board because it's happening. For example, going vegan–enjoy the ride family because I'm going to be happy or speaking Spanish. "Hola senorita" this is happening. If writing a book, ask them to turn the television volume down. Now don't be rude, but be clear and concise about what and why, and just ask for support and in return, you will support them in anything they want.

Got the time now to move. Now it's time to take action. There would be nothing worse than down to everyone, and then they berate you in your face for failing. Well, if it comes to that, then ask them to help you, ask them to support you in getting back to it. Ask them to do everything they can to help you find the time and whatever you need to get there. So, bring it back to the planning. What do you need? Do you need a laptop to write a book? Do you need audiobooks for learning a language? Do you need a book on how to set up and run a business? That last one is a key point. Do you need to spend the first few months learning how to do what you want to do? You may not even know where to start, so then learn it, get a book about it, and learn as much as you can. Speak to people that have done it.

In leveraging social media, you will easily be able to find people online that have done it and can easily drop them a message asking for advice. You want to work in a gym, then call a gym and speak to someone who is doing it, asking them everything you want to know. Maybe even go into one and ask them, how did they get there? What is good about it? What is bad about it? Once you have it laid out, then find as much additional time as you possibly can. Whatever the goal is, take it everywhere with you. Can you listen to audio versions of the books, videos online? Can you carry books, manuals, course work or whatever with you, in the car, in your locker at work? Can you use ten mins while on your break? Can you get up one hour earlier or just ten mins and spend time on it before anyone else gets up? You get up at four in the morning. The worst thing that will happen is you may be tired the next day. Now don't put yourself at risk with this if you are driving a lot the next day or operating a crane or something. Keep that in mind that preservation of you, your life and your family is the most important thing. Got an easy day, get up at four, you can go back to the power nap for 20 mins if needed. The key points here are to put you first on just that one thing, give yourself a great purpose and enjoy life a lot more, find what it is that you want and the benefit you will get. Plan it. Plan it some more and plan it again. Learn it if needed, everything you need to succeed.

Don't fear failure. If you fail, then work out why and then try again. But a key thing is, do you need to change your plan or your approach? I have a belief that most people in current times try for strive to perfection or to achieve a lot, and in which case, we put a lot of pressure on ourselves and a lot of stress. Remember to keep balance and to not overwork. I also think this belief probably comes from the media and competing with everyone else and, maybe even the messages we receive from our parents growing up or even our bosses at work– "Do this, don't do that. Stop it," and so on. Well, despite the purpose of this chapter and maybe even this book, maybe none of it really matters because you know what, no one is perfect, and no one will ever be perfect. So, stop worrying about it. I guess part of it might be a biological system that is in place to drive us to keep going and to strive to be better. Because if we didn't care at all, we probably wouldn't achieve anything. What we should really do is clear our minds from everything, set our own goals, and live our lives how we want to and try not to be too influenced by the outside world or even friends, family, and work colleagues. No more doing it for other people, do it for yourself. Now don't get me wrong here, you go to work for yourself to earn a living to live how you want, so then you may need to keep your boss happy. But you sure as hell don't need to kiss his ass. You can treat him like anyone else, like a friend or family member, talk about life and see what makes them tick, but don't treat them any different to your other colleagues. You can achieve anything you want. If you plan it, make time, take lots of small steps and some big steps to get there. Block out everything else and keep a balance to your life with rest when you need it, but not any more than that. Don't waste your time lying around watching television or phone scrolling if it's not your downtime. Plan that downtime or don't take it. Have the television on but, in the background, while you are working on your life mission, your goal, your dreams or whatever it is you want in life.

Chapter 10–Give It Away or Give to Others

I can remember as far back as being in school when a volunteer came in and did a talk about what they did and how they gave up their time for free. Now, as a teenager in school, I didn't quite get it. I didn't really have any reason to get it. I hadn't lived yet. After reading a book that covered a bit about giving back and the benefits, I came to realise it should be on my list, and then it was, and then I did. In doing so, I have come to learn a lot about other people and a lot about myself. It has also helped me to make the most of my time, as once a week I am giving up some time, which leaves me with even less time. So then, I make every effort not to waste any spare time that I have. Whether you decide to do something or not and whatever it is, then different opportunities will bring different benefits.

You have your dreams, your passions, your goals, and your vision. You have a plan. You have your finance in order. Your relationships are improving. Your diet is good. You're exercising. You may have taken massive action and you're living and working in a great place, clean, tidy and just how you want it. How do you feel? Are you happy or do you need something else? You may have gotten to a point in life where you have everything. Have you got to a point where you feel content? If you are lucky enough to have gotten to this place in life, then you may feel like life is okay, but not really exciting any more or that it lacks purpose or direction. Well, that can be dangerous. So, have you reviewed your plan, mission, values, etc. or have they just slipped? Are you finding it difficult to think of anything that you may want to work towards? Then think big. Make it so big that it is ridiculous, then go for it, it will give you great purpose and a great amount of work to do, so much so that it may even consume you. Then you will go from one extreme to the other.

Don't let any barriers get in your way. Don't let any negative beliefs stop you. As this will give you exactly what you desire and make your life so enjoyable and so rewarding. What about beyond that, what will give you great purpose and great fulfilment? You may be the only person that can answer that question. For me, what I have found and what I have learnt in life is that giving back and giving to others can really tick both those boxes, even if it's something you give back or give to people that benefit you too. Even better if that is the case, as it will keep you driven and motivated to do it more rather than doing it for the sake of it. For example, if you decide to have kids because you want to give life but then you do it for yourself as you want to have kids for your own personal reasons, there is mutual benefit and you really should be ticking both of those boxes before you proceed but you won't do much better in your life for creating purpose and fulfilment. How about charity work as another example? You could volunteer for an organisation to do some work for them, but if you don't get something out of it then, how will it give you purpose?

There is the simple element of it that it's rewarding, but I'm talking beyond that. I'm talking about being a little bit selfish and realising that there is more to be gained. It might be some sort of skill, some sort of training, or something you can use in your personal life. The more benefit you can get from it, the more you can give to them with regards to your time and commitment. If we were talking money, you could consider giving so much money to charity, be it monthly or in one-off payment, again consider the benefits to you. The more you can give, the more likely you will work to increase your income to be able to give more. Also, the more likely you will be able to find ways of earning more money to meet the demand for the extra money going out. The key thing, though, really is to consider how you are helping others and really the sense of purpose this will give your life. How will that help you in your personal life if you feel good about helping others? How will it help you with taking action, being motivated, learning to develop relationships, managing time, finance, achieving greatness and sustaining happiness? What would it be like if you took a few hours out of your week to do something for others rather than yourself, considering the majority of what we do is for ourselves and it doesn't always make us happy? Do you feel better when someone gives you something or when you give someone something? Either way, how long does that feeling last? Do you ever wonder why some of the richest people in the world, including royalty, take up charity work or give to charity? You could argue because they have the time and money. Sure, but what do they get out of it? They will get a good feeling of helping others, a sense of purpose and a sense of fulfilment. They will have something in their lives that gives them a real reason for being; something beyond themselves; something that will drive them forward motivate them to keep going.

Over the years, there have been some high profile, wealthy individuals that have suffered from anxiety, depression, self-harm and even taking their own lives. This clearly goes to show that success and money won't necessarily bring you happiness. So, it goes to show how important it is that you give purpose to your life if you're in a position where you feel like you may need it. Now, this may not be as far as helping others. It may just be the points at the start about missions, values, and goals. It will differ for everyone. The very least you can do if you are in a bad place is to try everything you can to get to a better place. You owe that much to yourself, your family, and your friends. It may be just using that brain of yours to learn and develop it beyond what you already know. It may be taking yourself away from everything by going on holiday, even if it's by yourself. That might even be the best option. The same concept goes really like the rest of the book– whatever works for you is probably the best option.

Try things out. If something works great, then keep going with it. If something doesn't work and you gave it a good chance and you tried it a few different ways, then move on and try something else. Whatever you do, make sure you realise your true purpose, your true sense of where you are going, in as many aspects of your life as possible. Realise that failure is just a part of life and when you fail on anything or even everything, it is just an opportunity to learn, including learning that you have to change your approach and go in a different direction for whatever it is, as this will help you to keep moving forward. Life is and always will be about you. There may be a time in life when it becomes about your kids, family, partner, and so on, but the key thing is that it is really and truly about you. Learn to like or even love yourself and find the things you like or love about yourself. We're always critical as it helps us to improve. That's fine, but don't let it get to the point of being unhealthy. Remember that there are good things about you too, even if you can't realise them. Work on it and find them. Don't let anyone tell you otherwise, and if people pay you a compliment, then take it.

Think about it. In your life, you might not have many people around you. You might not get out much and then you get out and help an organisation with their charity work. Then all of a sudden, you are out of the house, around people, and you have a great purpose to your life. One action could change your whole direction. You do have to focus on yourself. But sometimes changing your thought process and directing it to focus on others can really help you to change direction. Think outside the box and do things differently. If something isn't working, and life isn't great, how can you get there? Explore different options and do everything you can to get there. Give as much as you can and do for others as much as you can. Be a good person and reap the benefits of being a good person. Be smart. Don't let people take advantage of you. Do what's right and what is right for you and consider how you can help people while it also helps you. Take yourself forward to your funeral and think about how you want to be viewed by those people. How do you want people to talk about you when you are not in the room? How do you want to be remembered?

Chapter 11–Reflection, The Point to Life, Ups and Downs, and Knowing Yourself

I found my point to life after a few years of being lost. Once I found it, then the world changed for me. I have full focus and full direction. Everything else is just trivial. Like everyone, I have ups and downs, but at least now, I have more control over them, and I understand them. I accidentally came across the information about knowing yourself at an event I was attending and someone was talking about it. I didn't know I needed it but tried it anyway, as I am always curious about things like that. I found it to be extremely helpful to me in my life. I hope you find this of some benefit to yours.

Reflection, what is that? A person looking into a lake and seeing their face. You are staring in the mirror and really taking a look at yourself. Yes, a reflection of you. How do you see yourself? How do you want to see yourself? Just stop, pause, and take it in. Think about it for as long as you need to. What would your life be like if you chose how you really wanted it to be? Think about every element from your relationships to work to whatever is important to you. Why is it important to you? Take it beyond the superficial. Take it beyond the ridiculous dreams and bring it back to the real basics of life. Get all the real basics in place and then let the rest snowball. Make daily improvements to your life and daily goals. One small improvement in how you want life to be can really start to make your life a lot better. It can be anything; a small change in your diet, a daily walk, reaching out to someone you haven't spoken to in a while to build a bond and develop a relationship or reaching out to someone new.

How often do you make new friends or engage with someone different at work that you have never really spoken to? Why haven't you reached out to them? Where could they be in five years or even two? What could a bond with that person do for you when they have climbed the career ladder and you have a great working relationship? Make connections, make friends, even with your own family. How much do you talk? How much do you open up to your own family? Will they judge you? No, of course not. Will you challenge them on it if they do? Sure, you will. Reflect on everything in life–how your day has gone, how it could be better–and then write it down. What were your interactions like? What responses did you get? How can you change your communication to get better responses? What do you want from people? What do you want from your life?

You feel down and you feel high/up. Yes, that happens. Why? It could be a range of things. It could be sugar or caffeine in your diet, it could be an experience or emotion, it could be hormone related, or it could be exercise, weather, and/or people around you. A whole list of things out in the world that could affect how you feel. Are you aware of what is causing you to feel the way you do? Do you have any control over any of these things? Can you affect all of them? Sure, you can manage them, once you know what they are and what makes it better for you. Do you find it best to maintain a steady balance, as being up for some time is only going to lead to one thing? Yes, you know the answer, crashing back down. Make a log, a daily diary of how you feel. Record three times a day– morning, after lunch and after dinner; happy, sad, tired, bored, miserable, depressed, suicidal, amazing, or whatever it may be. Record other information, such as what you have eaten, what you have been doing, what you believe caused those feelings. Do it for as long as you can–three days, a week, four weeks; as much as possible. Then look back over it for patterns.

What can you do to manage your feelings and your mood? Can you make minor changes to your diet, alcohol intake, caffeine, high-sugar foods, or even the opposite? You may be feeling tired and not consuming much sugar or carbohydrates. Are you feeling tired because you have been to the gym every night for the last two weeks? You get the idea. Once you have a clear and simple guide to what is causing your mood, you can start to put a change in place to improve your feelings. It might even be the people you spend time with. But once you know, you can implement the changes. You can then even continue to log for the following few weeks or even more, and then see if the changes are helping, and if not, then you could make more changes and keep going until you have a solid balance to your life with a nice steady level of wellbeing and mindset with very little external factors affecting you. It might even be that you went to bed too late, so got up too late and then got caught in traffic and ended up late for work, which caused you a lot of stress. Quite simple. But think back to why you went to bed late. Was it your routine? Was it seeking pleasure from something, avoiding pain in some way? Most of what we do as people is either to seek pleasure or avoid pain. Something worth thinking about for any of your actions in life and why you do the things you do in life.

The point of life is an interesting aspect and a question that will forever be upon us. I do have a strong belief that the answer is different for everyone in the same way. What is your ideal weight, or what is your favourite colour? I believe rather than the question being what is the point of life; I believe what is the point of your life should be the question. In which case it comes back to you; only you know that answer to the question, what is the point of your life? Now, you may not know the answer. That doesn't mean there isn't a point to your life. That means you haven't found out the answer yet. A bit like not really knowing how much you would like your ideal weight to be. You might need some guidance. You might need someone to tell you what a good weight is to be. So then, it could be the same. You might need someone to tell you a range of things you could do with your life. Right, so someone could give you ideas, but unless that person cares about it as much as you, they may not put much effort into helping you; so, it is on you. It's as easy as picking up your phone and going online and spending some time researching it or even better, lie on your bed, close your eyes, block out the world and think about life and how you want it to be and what the ideal life for you would be. Do everything and do as much as you can to find the answer.

Find what the point is of your life, give yourself a purpose, learn as much as you can, however you can, even if it's through YouTube videos. Learn about everything you need to learn about to help. You find what will give you a great purpose when you find it. I assure you that you will find it. If you can get this far in a book, then you can. You will be the sort of person that won't give up on your purpose. Once you get there when you find it, the point of your life, the purpose, I want you to realise that it is not the be-all or end-all of your life.

Nothing in life is permanent, including your purpose. Your purpose can be reviewed daily, weekly, monthly, or yearly. Whatever you want whenever you want. This is so important, as it will need to change. As you grow and develop as a person, then your life and purpose will change. Even as you age, your purpose at 20 years old may be different when you get to 40 years old. Also, think about how it could affect you. If your purpose was to have a family with your partner and then your partner left you, then your life's purpose would have been crushed and it may leave you in a bad place. So, try to make your purpose flexible, maybe have as much detail as possible but with great freedom, for it to move and change. Your partner may have left but it may change to meeting someone new. Sometimes you have to take a step sideways to move forward, to get around that wall. Maybe even have more than one purpose and consider more than one way of achieving your purpose for each one. Whatever it is, and whatever you want, whatever makes you happy, spend some of your time on it. Do you spend more time per day on the toilet then on your life's purpose? Do you spend more time doing something for someone else than your life's purpose? Do you spend more time stuck in traffic or more time queuing at a checkout? You get my point and now surely you realise that is completely ridiculous. At the very least, you should be spending a similar amount of time each day just writing down what you want in life and what the purpose of your life is. Maybe even just sitting down thinking about it and maybe even just reviewing it. How will doing this change your life? Will this small little action of maybe ten minutes in the morning make you feel so much better about life? Will it make you feel so much better about your day ahead? Will it make you feel like you have direction, and will it make you feel like you have a purpose, a passion, and even a life? Will it make you feel alive and will it keep you alive?

Knowing yourself: What good is all this, if you don't even know who you are. Establishing your values and mission will certainly help, but what about understanding the reasons why you do things differently than others and how you act and behave. How can you utilise your characteristics to your benefit, so that you can excel in whatever it is you want to do? There are multiple ways of finding out who you really are, maybe even starting with a bit of self-reflection on what makes you tick, what drives you, and how events in your life have shaped you and affected you. There is also a test you can do, one of many different variants called the Myers-Briggs type indicator. This can be accessed online, and you go through a range of questions to identify your personality type (there should be free versions online as well as paid). The personality type that you get is one of 16 and it will give you a breakdown, including an introduction, strengths and weakness, relationships, friendship, parenthood, career, and a conclusion. Once you have the breakdown, then you can read through and learn things about yourself that you may already know but didn't quite realise or know why you were like that or why you do certain things. It will then give you a clear understanding which you can use to help in your life, and even more so, it may help you to realise that there is nothing wrong with the way that you are and that everyone is different in some way. You don't have to be perfect and no one ever will be, but you sure as hell can try, work, strive and fight to be number one because you deserve it.

Summary

To summarise and to get across to you the key point, meaning and purpose of this book. The aim is to provide you the reader with a tangible product that can help you to improve your life and in a range of areas. Be it be small changes or big changes. I wanted to share the things I have learned from reading and life experiences. To help you with your personal development and growth.

I have tried to cover a wide range of areas and I am sure I could have added more, but didn't want to go to off track. I also didn't want to dilute the content. The key message within the book is for you to focus on yourself, to look after yourself. To be the best you can be for you, your family and friends. To find and live a happy life regardless of all the struggles you will face.

I would say that I want you to come away from this with a good balance to your life. A clear direction or realisation that you should have a purpose and do everything you can to find it and live it. For you to realise that you're important and that you can do great things for you and for others. You can become a well-rounded individual with good health, good people around you. You can make your life and living conditions whatever you want them to be. You can take full control over everything.

Whatever happens in your life, whatever has happened? The key thing to focus on is having a great time and living as much of your life as you can. Be happy, laugh and joke and make sure you do it every day.

I hide no fact this is my first book and I know the edit isn't perfect by any means. I got to the point that I would rather release the book being imperfect than not release it. The key thing for me was getting the message out so that I can help you or whoever needs it. I have also learnt from the experience and it will help me to make sure any books I write will be free from errors.

I hope it helps you and anyone that is close to you. If you have gained any benefit this book, then please share it. I would love to hear about your steps towards greatness and happiness. Thank you for reading and I hope you have a great life.

The End

About the Author

After writing my first two books, which were non-
fiction. Based around areas of knowledge and expertise.
I gained throughout my working career and through
further research. I decided to have a go at writing a
novel, something I always dreamed of doing.
Throughout the process, I discovered my love of writing
fiction. This led to self-publishing my books and
completing every process, from editing to cover design. I
continue to this day as an independent author. Writing
alongside working full-time, parenting and volunteering.
Along with the other challenges of life.

My main focus is to give as much as I can and to help as
many people as possible I can. Give people stories to
pull them away from the normality of their day. But
most important to enjoy every step. If any of my books
or work have helped you or if you have enjoyed them, I
would love to hear about it. As that it what makes it so
enjoyable. Thank you.

For more information visit

Contact: BenjaminHarris@gmx.com